Praise for *The*

"It is impossible to express in a few lines the breadth and depth of this remarkable book. In *The Way of Virtue*, Robert Peng has brought to life those ancient Daoist and Buddhist teachings that can transform our understanding and way of being in the world. He writes with an accessible simplicity that lays out a profound map of spiritual insight and invites us to engage with life-changing practices that have borne fruit for thousands of years. His many examples are incisively apt, often expressed with a lightness and humor that captivates the reader. It's rare to come across a book that is so comprehensive in its scope, so practical in its application, and so inspiring in its effect. Highly recommended for anyone wishing to explore for themselves the great illuminating mystery of Dao."

JOSEPH GOLDSTEIN
author of *Mindfulness*

"It is not surprising that the classic of Daoism is called The Classic of the Way and Its Virtue, because it is, after all, virtue and behavior that reveal our philosophy of life and allow us to be of service in the world. Robert Peng's *The Way of Virtue* is an expression of this great truth. His book masterfully intertwines ethics and Daoist wisdom, providing tangible and practical insights into everyday life. The inclusion of transformative practices like the Wogu hand seal, the Ong Ahh Hong chant, and nuanced descriptions of Healing Sounds enriches the narrative, making it a compelling read. Whether you are new to Asian healing arts or an experienced practitioner, *The Way of Virtue* will inspire and guide you to a new level of understanding and vibrant well-being."

KENNETH COHEN
author of *The Way of Qigong*

"*The Way of Virtue* teaches meditation that goes beyond the mind and leads into the wisdom of the body. It teaches us how to awaken the Spirit and reengage the world from this awakened space. I particularly loved the journey Robert Peng takes his readers on through the wisdom of the meridians. I highly recommend this masterpiece to everyone, from the novice to the experienced seeker."

DONNA EDEN
author of *Energy Medicine*

"Robert Peng, a master of Qigong, shares his deep understanding of this spiritual art with us in *The Way of Virtue*. This is a marvelous guide in the universal journey of awakening."

DANIEL GOLEMAN, PHD
author of *Emotional Intelligence*

"Robert Peng brilliantly illuminates a path through a profound ancient healing wisdom tradition. In a clear, insightful, and accessible way, he adapts Qigong principles to modern life challenges and shares the common sense of virtue for our lives and the world."

TARA BENNETT-GOLEMAN
author of *Emotional Alchemy*

"If you're longing to explore the profound mystery of existence, asking 'Who am I?' and 'Why are we here?' this book is for you. Poetic and practical, *The Way of Virtue* serves as your guide on the journey to greater peace. Robert Peng and Rafael Nasser blend philosophy, soulful stories, and meditation practices, leading readers through a step-by-step awakening along the Daoist path with Buddhist insights. This book is a supportive friend that will help you experience greater emptiness and wholeness with each breath."

SHARON SALZBERG
author of *Lovingkindness* and *Real Life*

"Robert Peng is a genius at distilling esoteric Daoist practices into practical, useful, and accessible teachings for everyday life. The world is calling for more virtue—living with a compassionate, kind heart. This book is truly the way to virtuous living. Use this wisdom as a guide to embodying ancient practices for a happy, healthy, fulfilling modern life."

LEE HOLDEN
author, producer, TV personality, and Qigong Master

The
WAY of VIRTUE

Other books by Robert Peng and Rafael Nasser:

The Master Key: Qigong Secrets for Vitality, Love, and Wisdom

The
WAY of VIRTUE

Qigong Meditations to Cultivate
Perfect Peace in an Imperfect World

ROBERT PENG

with Rafael Nasser

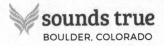
sounds true
BOULDER, COLORADO

Sounds True
Boulder, CO

This book is not intended as a substitute for the medical recommendations of physicians, mental health professionals, or other health-care providers. Rather, it is intended to offer information to help the reader cooperate with physicians, mental health professionals, and health-care providers in a mutual quest for optimal well-being. We advise readers to carefully review and understand the ideas presented and to seek the advice of a qualified professional before attempting to use them.

Published 2024

Book design by Meredith Jarrett

Cover design and interior illustrations by Tobin Dorn

Interior photographs by Evan Lui and Ramon Fernandez

Cover photo by Ramon Fernandez

Models for the illustrations: Alejandra Cohen, Ishmael Cato, and Ellen Petersen

Printed in Canada

BK06740

Library of Congress Cataloging-in-Publication Data

Names: Peng, Robert, author. | Nasser, Rafael, author.
Title: The way of virtue : Qigong meditations to cultivate perfect peace in an imperfect world / Robert Peng with Rafael Nasser.
Description: Boulder, CO : Sounds True, 2024.
Identifiers: LCCN 2023040850 (print) | LCCN 2023040851 (ebook) | ISBN 9781649631510 (trade paperback) | ISBN 9781649631527 (ebook)
Subjects: LCSH: Qi gong. | Meditation--Therapeutic use.
Classification: LCC RA781.8 .P463 2024 (print) | LCC RA781.8 (ebook) |
DDC 613.7/1489--dc23/eng/20240118
LC record available at https://lccn.loc.gov/2023040850
LC ebook record available at https://lccn.loc.gov/2023040851

FSC
www.fsc.org
MIX
Paper | Supporting
responsible forestry
FSC® C016245

Dedicated to Laozi (Lao Tzu), the founder of Daoism

Table of Contents

List of Exercises

 Audio recordings of the healing sounds and detailed images of the energy points referenced in the exercises can be found at robertpeng.com/six-healing-sounds-images.

Introduction

I was born in Xiangtan, China, during the Cultural Revolution. Xiangtan was a bustling industrial city that centered on a large steel factory. My parents worked at the factory, and we lived across the street from a gated compound that hosted dignitaries and government officials that visited the factory. I was an eight-year-old boy and I liked to sneak into the compound to explore the colorful gardens and fruit trees that contrasted vividly with the utilitarian gray concrete buildings that surrounded it. One day, I discovered the boiler room that generated the hot water that was piped throughout the compound. I peered in through the open door and I was mesmerized by the fiery furnaces. Mr. Tan, the boiler room attendant, saw me and invited me inside. He was a kind man, and we watched the fire together. We became friends that day and I would visit him regularly. He seemed to appreciate my company.

Mr. Tan was a senior monk from a mountain monastery that had been disbanded by the authorities. In those days, religion was viewed as incompatible with the revolutionary ideals of the times, and the remote mountaintop monastery was shuttered. As a monk, Mr. Tan was known as Xiao Yao, which means "easy going." He embodied the meaning of his name. His presence brought me a sense of peace that I had never experienced with anyone else. In his presence, the complications of life dissolved and I experienced serenity. After spending some time together in the boiler room, Xiao Yao revealed that he knew martial arts and offered to teach me. This was a risky proposition because the government authorities shunned any form of classical Chinese culture, including the martial arts. I enthusiastically agreed to become his secret student with the blessing of my parents.

Before too long, I realized that Xiao Yao possessed unusual abilities both as a martial artist and a healer. He was an accomplished monk who had spent his entire life cultivating his body, mind, and spirit. As I grew to know him better, he became my spiritual master and guided me toward exalted experiences that defied my imagination. I became a devoted disciple who practiced martial arts and meditation diligently several hours a day before and after school.

When I was a teenager, government policies were relaxed, and Xiao Yao's monastery reopened. He returned to manage the repair of the derelict structures, and while I was willing to follow him back, he instructed me to complete my studies and to join him on my winter and summer breaks. When I was fifteen years old, I arrived at the monastery ready to practice with him as we always had in Xiangtan. But instead, he informed me that I would be spending my summer break in a dark chamber below the main temple hall fasting and meditating for one hundred days. I had been meditating for years and I trusted Xiao Yao with my life. I followed him into the dark chamber. He gave me instructions and left me alone. Every day he returned to burn an incense stick. The glow acclimated my eyes to the light. He brought me fresh water and taught me new meditations. Then he would leave again.

Days passed and blurred into weeks. My meditations deepened. I was transforming spiritually, and one day, everything changed. I entered a state of consciousness traditionally known as *Small Death Big Life*. My pulse slowed down and became imperceptible. I barely breathed. Had anyone stumbled on me in that state, I would have appeared to be dead. But inwardly, I was teeming with the essence of eternity. I remained in this state of suspended animation, dissolved into the radiance of the Supreme Ultimate, for eight days. I might have remained in that state indefinitely, but Xiao Yao reeled me back into my embodied state of consciousness. Gradually, I became myself again, but everything had transformed. I had awakened a sublime sense of self, new healing gifts, and divine blessings. I experienced myself anew and related to the world with profound reverence.

My hundred-day adventure in the dark chamber was the culmination of a spiritual process that had unfolded over various stages of development. The book that you are holding, *The Way of Virtue*, is an introduction to the meditation practices that prepared me for the dark chamber. The book is divided into two parts. Part 1, Aspects of Mind, presents a Qigong theory of mind that sets the stage for part 2, The Journey to Spirit, which includes three meditation practices designed to elicit the direct experience of your true nature.

What is the taste of chocolate? The clearest way to answer the question is to taste chocolate. The second-best way to answer the question is to smell the aroma of chocolate. The aroma is a lesser experience than the taste, but it gets us closer to a meaningful answer than an abstract description made up of words. What is your true nature? The clearest way to answer the question is to "taste" your true nature. For most people, that experience requires a committed meditation practice. The book you hold in your hands is a guide that can lead you toward experience. A simpler, though less complete way to answer the question, is to imbibe the "aroma" of your true nature. We can prompt that experience right now by reflecting on a series of questions that invoke the palpable mystery of being human.

A series of primal questions shadow each one of us every moment of every day. Who am I? Why do I exist? Who are you? Why does anything exist? What is *really* going on? On most days we wake up, shower, brush our teeth, get dressed, eat, commute, work, eat, work, socialize, eat, watch television, shower, sleep, and cycle through some variation of this routine. Throughout our waking hours we focus on deadlines and workflows, we are distracted by news and gossip, we delight in food and pleasure, we are drawn into the dramas on our phones, we fight, we kiss, we play, we exercise, we live our lives. All the while, the primal questions hover over us like unnoticed clouds every ticking second of the day.

Occasionally, the natural order subverts, and our lives fall through the cracks of clock time into the abyss of chaos. We unexpectedly lose a loved one, we bump elbows with mortality, we witness horror that disrupts the rhythm of our daily routine, and the primal questions come into sharp view. Who am I? Why do I exist? Who are you? Why does anything exist? What is *really* going on? As you stumble over these questions sincerely and with an open heart, you are within proximity of the "aroma" of your true nature. Pursuing those questions through reflection and meditation can lead us to the direct apprehension of our true nature, our Spirit. But more often, we attempt to quell the sting of the primal questions by turning to religion or science. However, both faith and reason remain mute in the face of the primal questions. God is an unknowable mystery, and the laws of physics break down at the edge of space-time. What preceded Creation? What preceded the Big Bang? Who or what set the Universe in motion and why? Ask a priest and a scientist and they will both shrug in unison. The primal questions cannot be answered by words, metaphors, stories, theories, facts, or formulas. The only way to answer them meaningfully is to pursue a mystical path that leads the mind back to the undifferentiated center of your being. When you experience your mind as unified and perfectly peaceful, the unequivocal realization of your true nature as Spirit dawns organically.

Envision our Universe as an expanding circle. The center point of this circle, also known as the Origin, symbolizes the unknowable root of all things. Somehow, the Origin of all things radiated outward and the titanic trio of space-time, matter, and energy manifested. Subatomic particles came into being as the circle expanded. Subatomic particles gave rise to atoms. The circle expanded again. Atoms gave rise to molecules, molecules to cells, cells to aquatic life, aquatic life to amphibians, reptiles, mammals, monkeys and apes, hominids, archaic humans, and archaic humans—through a series of momentous cultural leaps—evolved tribal, horticultural, agricultural, industrial, and digital cultures and technologies. Each stage of this evolutionary spiral enveloped the preceding stages and with every developmental whirl, each evolving entity expanded in breadth of experience, depth of feeling, and height of intelligence.

Modern and postmodern human beings represent the pinnacle of this evolutionary process. We stand at the outermost edge of the circle on our planet. Despite the remarkable progress we made as a species, the problems that plague our planet appear to have grown in proportion to our achievements. The threat of violence continues to hang over personal, interpersonal, communal, and international relations. Mental health problems are sweeping across entire populations in record numbers. Economic swings undermine our sense of stability and rattle social cohesion. Climate change and disease threaten our well-being. Nuclear weapons threaten every heartbeat on the planet.

Imagine scrunching all the suffering of every human being into a ball and scrunching all the well-being of every human being into another ball and placing those two balls on a scale. Which way does the scale tip? Unfortunately, progress does not appear to be correlated to contentment and technological development is not a substitute for peace. Despite improved life conditions, a general state of malcontent characterizes the human condition.

In Asia around twenty-five hundred years ago, two teachers emerged as beacons of spiritual wisdom: Buddha and Laozi (or Lao Tzu.) These noble souls proclaimed to possess the knowledge to redress the malcontent inherent in the human experience. Both teachers had a common message: by returning to the mysterious Origin of all things that lies within each one of us we can quell the primal questions of existence, end existential suffering, and experience genuine peace.

The disciples of Buddha who returned to the Origin and attained Nirvana became known as Bodhisattvas. The disciples of Laozi who returned to the Origin and reunited with the eternal Dao became known as Immortals. Both Bodhisattvas and Immortals traveled inwardly through meditation to the Origin of all things and awakened Perfect Peace. That inner process defines the journey to Spirit. The word "Spirit" refers to a unified mind grounded in perfect peace that arises effortlessly from within and offers boundless virtues to an imperfect world. Imagine waking up from the most restful sleep on the most beautiful morning. In the twilight of peaceful sleep, we sometimes experience a fleeting sense of unified well-being. That state approximates the deep inner contentment that arises when we awaken our spiritual nature. Imagine being able to pursue your daily affairs soundly immersed in an imperturbable sense of well-being. You would still experience mundane thoughts and emotions, but those experiences would ebb and flow like gentle waves in a peaceful ocean of tranquility.

Xiao Yao embodied that quality of peace in the face of the greatest adversity. He taught his disciples the way to peace through meditation. The amalgamation of Buddhism and Daoism is commonplace in Chinese spirituality and the method he taught me to awaken Spirit is like the Daoist method traditionally known as Internal Alchemy or Neidan (ney-dan). But he never used those terms and his version deviates from some of the other teachings I read about many years later, so I will avoid using those terms as well. Xiao Yao dwelt on theory and scripture sparingly. He did not fuss over names, words, symbols, or stories that distracted from the goal of direct experience.

Xiao Yao's spiritual method does not require any beliefs on the part of a practitioner. Maybe you adhere to a religion or maybe you shun religion altogether. Everyone can undergo the spiritual journey regardless of their religious affiliation or beliefs. The prerequisite for a successful spiritual journey is the sincere desire to awaken the fundamental essence of your being. This desire transcends any belief.

In *The Way of Virtue,* I present the teachings of Xiao Yao in the simplest way so that it can be a guide to the greatest number of people of as many backgrounds as possible. Practice diligently and you will also advance toward perfection and awaken your virtue. Virtue is the litmus test of your spiritual condition. With each stride that you take toward perfection, a more refined kind of virtue arises. Three meditations are taught in the *Way of Virtue*. Each meditation awakens a particular aspect of mind and a related virtue. The Six Healing Sounds awakens Higher Mind and goodwill, the Twelve Meridian Empowerment awakens Pure Mind and benevolence, and Huo Lu Gong awakens Spirit and peace.

The sixteenth chapter of the Dao De Jing—*The Classic Work (Jing) on the Virtue (De) of the Way (Dao)*—which is attributed to Laozi, distills Daoist wisdom to a single cryptic sentence, "Going back to the Origin is called peace." This book is a guide that transforms the meaning of these words into a series of practical steps.

The meditation practices presented in *The Way of Virtue* require patience, discipline, and habitual repetition. Master one exercise before moving on to the next. Savor the process. Reflect on your progress. Delight in the experience, and as you become a more refined version of yourself, channel the well-being you cultivate into your words and actions. Strive to transform your life into a blessing for the world.

Like all adventures, the journey to Spirit begins with a first step. In our case, that step involves exploring some basic concepts presented in my first book, *The Master Key.*

Part 1

ASPECTS OF MIND

1

Basic Concepts

The Three Dantians and the Central Meridian

Everybody that is born dies. One moment a heart is beating, a chest is rising and falling, eyes are blinking, and the next moment, life departs, and we are standing before an inert object.

In Daoism, the distance between life and death is measured in terms of Qi (chee) energy. Qi is a broad term that can be compared to electricity. Run electricity through a bulb and it lights up. Run electricity through a satellite phone and you can communicate with anyone anywhere on the surface of the planet. The same electrical current powers a vacuum cleaner and a blower. Likewise, Qi powers the myriad functions related to our internal organs and our cells. Qi regulates digestion and respiration, circulation, and excretion. All our vital functions reflect the quality of our Qi flow. When Qi is running properly through our body, we are alive and thrive. When Qi flow is imbalanced or deficient, symptoms of ill health arise. When Qi flow stops, we die. Qi is synonymous with life force.

Daoist masters mapped out the major routes of Qi flow inside the human body with exquisite precision. Perhaps you have seen an acupuncture chart punctuated with hundreds of energy points running along a dozen meridian lines. Those charts represent some of the main channels that Qi follows. The points serve unique functions, and regulating them through acupuncture or Qigong meditation allows us to divert life force from one part of the body to another. That concept is central to Chinese medicine and self-cultivation. Daoist masters also mapped out three energy centers that are more fundamental, though less familiar, than the meridians and the acupuncture points. These energy centers, known as the Three Dantians (dan-tee-yen), are interlinked by a powerful central channel known as the Central Meridian. This network of energy centers forms the backbone of the human energy system, and developing an awareness of the Three Dantians and the Central Meridian defines the starting point of our journey.

Please look at Figure 1.1 below.

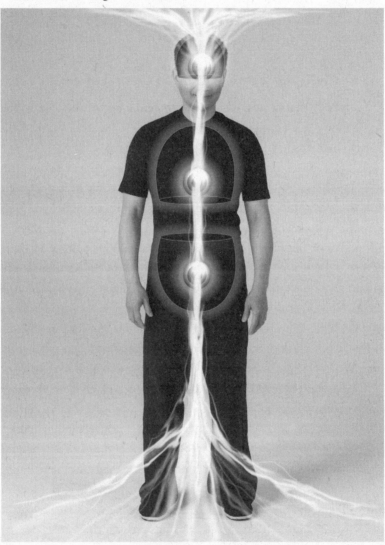

Figure 1.1: Dantian and the Central Meridian

Notice the three spherical energy centers. Each of these is a Dantian and can be envisioned as a little sun radiating Qi energy from its core. When you awaken and empower the three Dantians, you literally feel an energy vibration radiating from the center and filling your body with warmth and a sense of well-being.

Each Dantian is associated with a specific quality. The Upper Dantian is the energy field located at the center of the head. This center regulates wisdom and creative intelligence. Imagine having to decide between two jobs and being intuitively guided toward one over the other. You envision one option working out better. While you can't prove that decision is the right one, you are guided inwardly. When the Upper Dantian is radiating healthy Qi, we feel guided and tend to make better life choices. And when the Upper Dantian is blocked or deficient, we are unable to feel guided or envision the way forward. We feel as disoriented as a spinning compass needle and we lack a trustworthy sense of direction. The Upper Dantian is associated with Wisdom.

The Middle Dantian is the sphere located in the center of the chest cavity behind the sternum. This center regulates the capacity for love and compassion. Imagine your heart opening in the presence of someone you love. You feel deep warmth and tenderness emanating from the center of your chest. When the Middle Dantian is awakened and radiating healthy Qi, you experience open-hearted love toward people close to you and compassion toward strangers. Love is a spectrum that extends from the personal to the universal, and as the Middle Dantian develops, so does our capacity to love the world. When the Middle Dantian is blocked or deficient, our capacity to love is brittle and, in some cases, the heart shuts down and becomes a beating stone unable to give or receive any love at all.

The Lower Dantian is the sphere located slightly below the navel in the lower abdomen. This center regulates sexual energy and our ability to act in the world. Imagine waking up in the morning overflowing with vitality. You push through the day like a workhorse full of drive. When the Lower Dantian is awakened and empowered, our capacity for endurance increases. You feel vital and alive and are rearing to go like a racehorse about to start a race. When the Lower Dantian is blocked or deficient, getting out of bed just to feed yourself feels like a daunting task. When a menial task feels like carrying a sack of rocks up a steep hill, our Lower Dantian is probably depleted.

Wisdom, Love, and Vitality define the functions of the three fundamental centers of our energy body. These three centers are integrated by an energy channel called the Central Meridian that runs from the top of the head to the perineum and interpenetrates the Three Dantians. The Central Meridian extends above the head to connect with celestial energies and below the pelvic floor to connect with the energies of the earth.

The Central Meridian regulates our Wisdom, Love, and Vitality. When the Central Meridian is in a state of flow and connected to the earth and the sky, our Wisdom, Love, and Vitality are expressed in an integrated way. Such an individual experiences Wisdom rooted in Love, Love rooted in Vitality, and Vitality rooted in Wisdom. When you encounter a person with a Central Meridian streaming healthy Qi, you are in the presence an integrated human being.

When the Central Meridian is deficient or unable to flow freely, we may feel Wisdom, Love, and Vitality at different times in different situations, but we lack the ability to experience all those qualities simultaneously. Imagine a wise woman who can't connect her creative energies to her Vitality. She lacks the power to convert her intuition into action. Or an athlete who lacks the capacity to integrate sexual Vitality with Love. Or a big-hearted friend who cares deeply but offers terrible guidance.

My teacher, Xiao Yao, referred to the Three Dantians and the Central Meridian as the Four Golden Wheels. "Golden" refers to the happiness these energy centers provide when they are circulating Qi as an integrated unit. Happiness that relies on the gratification of the senses is a temporary fix. And while there is inherently nothing wrong with enjoying the fruits of the world, we cannot sustain happiness when we depend on pleasure for our well-being. The Four Golden Wheels generate organic happiness that is self-sustaining and arises from within.

The exercises in my first book, *The Master Key*, are designed to systematically awaken and empower the Four Golden Wheels. The following exercise draws on some of the practices described in that book to help you awaken these energy centers. But before we can begin to practice, we need to learn how to sit properly for meditation practice. Adopting the Natural Sitting Posture is essential to all the exercises presented in this book.

Exercise 1: Effortless Sitting

Sit comfortably on the floor, on a meditation cushion, or on a chair. Do not try to look like a monk seated in full lotus position if crossing your legs constricts blood flow or causes any kind of discomfort. Discomfort will distract your attention while you meditate. Sitting comfortably while maintaining structural alignment is important. Proper structure is emphasized for the practices taught in this book because we often use chanting to activate our internal organs, and the proper alignment of the spine transforms our torso into a resonance chamber. When we are sitting properly, we become like an auditorium with good acoustics. We can chant a sound and direct that vibration to a specific part of the body. If we slump or lean back, we dampen the sound and the vibration does not reach its destination.

When you are sitting, allow the natural curvature of your spine to keep the vertebrae stacked on top of each other. Avoid slumping over or resting on a wall or the back of the chair. When your spine and the soft tissues surrounding the vertebrae are properly aligned, each vertebra will hold up the weight of all the others above it without muscular strain. The sacrum supports the lumbar vertebrae, the lumbar vertebrae support the thoracic vertebrae, and the thoracic vertebrae support the cervical vertebrae that extend into the base of your skull.

Once you are seated comfortably, rest your hands on your lap in a relaxed position. Keep your hands positioned comfortably so that they do not strain and divert your attention from the meditation.

Whether you are seated on the ground or a chair, feel the weight of your body transferring through the ischial tuberosities, your sitz bones. If you are sitting on a chair, feel that weight travel through your legs to your feet. Feel yourself rooted to the ground through the soles of your feet.

To summarize, your vertebrae are stacked without requiring muscular effort. Your arms and shoulders are comfortable and relaxed without muscular strain. Your body's weight extends to the floor through your sitz bones and through your feet if you are sitting on a chair.

When you are seated properly, you quickly lose your body sense. The structural integrity formed by your skeletal alignment dissolves the burden of weight. When you are properly aligned, your breathing is effortless. Your organs hang comfortably like fruits on a tree without feeling any internal pressure. By simply adopting Natural Sitting Posture, you automatically enter a deeply relaxed and meditative state.

Once you are seated comfortably, close your eyes. Feel your lids touching gently and allow the tip of your tongue to rest comfortably against the largest groove you encounter on your upper palate. The tongue will wedge and rest effortlessly in that position. Feel your tongue relaxed and steady. This is the natural tongue resting position. Breathe naturally through your nose, inhaling and exhaling effortlessly. Do not control the breath. This is called natural breathing.

Spinal alignment with eyes closed, natural tongue resting position, and natural breathing position establish the Natural Sitting Posture. With most of the exercises in this book, I begin with the words, "Adopt Natural Sitting Posture." All the details described above are implied by that phrase.

1. Sit comfortably on a chair, a meditation cushion, or the floor.

2. Feel your sacrum, lumbar spine, thoracic spine, and cervical spine form an integrated structure.

3. Trace the alignment of each vertebra from the top of your spine to the sacrum.

4. Feel the weight of your body travel down your spine to your hips and your sitz bones. If you are seated on a chair, feel the weight of your legs root to the ground through your feet.

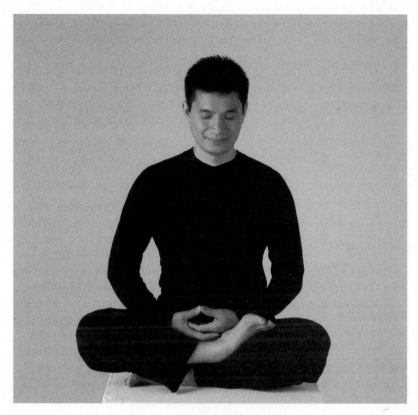

Figure 1.2: Natural Sitting Posture

5. Rest your forearms comfortably on your thighs. Clasp your hands or keep them on your lap. Relax your hands and your fingers. Your hand position should be free of tension or strain.

6. Place your tongue on the first groove of your upper palate.

7. Breathe naturally through your nose.

8. Close your eyes.

9. You are now in Natural Sitting Posture. Breath naturally for three cycles or more and open your eyes.

Exercise 2: Chanting Ong, Ahh, Hong

Now that you are familiar with Natural Sitting Posture, we can introduce an exercise that uses sound vibration to awaken the Four Golden Wheels. Sound vibration is a useful meditation tool because it penetrates internally. While you can easily massage an acupuncture point on your arm, you can't poke your finger through your ear and massage the center of your head. However, you can activate the center of your head using the sound, ONG. ONG is the sound of the Upper Dantian. In this exercise, we adopt Natural Sitting Posture and chant ONG repeatedly, *ongggg . . . ongggg . . . ongggg . . .* We pause between chants to feel the vibration at the center of your head.

Next, we chant the sound of the Middle Dantian, AHH. Chant AHH out loud a few times, *ahhhhh . . . ahhhhh . . . ahhhhh . . .* Direct the vibration to the center of your chest toward the Middle Dantian.

Next, intone the sound of the Lower Dantian—located at the center of your lower abdomen slightly below and behind your navel— HONG. *Honggg . . . honggg . . . honggg . . .* Direct the vibration toward the Lower Dantian.

Finally, we combine all three sounds to activate the Central Meridian. Inhale and become aware of the sky above your head. Chant: ONG, AHH, HONG and feel the vibration flow along the Center Meridian, the central axis of your body. When you end the chant, bring your awareness to the ground below you, and as you inhale, become aware of the sky again and chant: ONG, AHH, HONG. Below you will find the formal instructions for this exercise.

1. Adopt the Natural Sitting Posture.

2. Inhale and become aware of the sky above your head.

3. Chant ONG, AHH, HONG. Feel the sound vibration awaken your Upper, Middle, and Lower Dantians. *Ongggg . . . ahhhhh . . . honggg . . .* Repeat nine or more times.

4. When you complete the chant, become aware of the earth.

5. Repeat the chant nine times or more.

6. Sit silently for nine breaths or more and open your eyes.

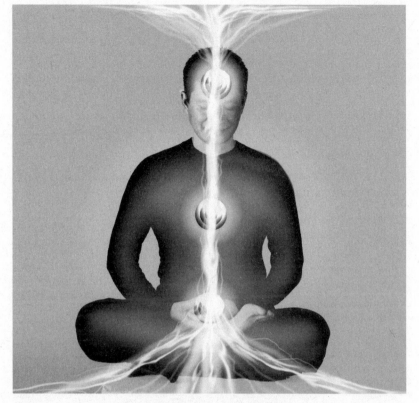

Figure 1.3: Chanting Ong, Ahh, Hong

Exercise 3: Nourish Your Qi

After we finish meditating, we Nourish your Qi. This is a practice that we use to close every exercise. We can compare mediation practice to making tea. First, we heat up the water, and then we steep the tea. Steeping the tea is like nourishing our Qi. It is a passive activity. We do nothing. The lack of action *is* the action. Every practice activates our energy body. After we end the activity, we allow our body to simmer in an ocean of Universal Qi, the background energy of the Universe. We envision ourselves as a sponge immersed in water. Is the sponge inside the water or is the water inside the sponge? Both are true. My master, Xiao Yao, would describe Nourishing Qi as, *"I am in Qi; Qi is in me."*

Begin by sitting or lying comfortably. Make sure the floor does not feel cold or hard. Feel yourself floating in an endless expanse of energy that is illuminated and bright, as bright as if the sun were shining directly overhead and radiating though the water. *I am in Qi; Qi is in me.* Allow this energy to nourish your body. Every cell in your body is soaking in Universal Qi. You are becoming brighter and lighter. *I am in Qi; Qi is in me.* You are dissolving into a beautiful ocean. This ocean is endless and boundless and you are basking in the warmth of the light. *I am in Qi; Qi is in me.* Nourish your Qi. Allow yourself to become light and bright, endless and boundless, until your eyes open naturally.

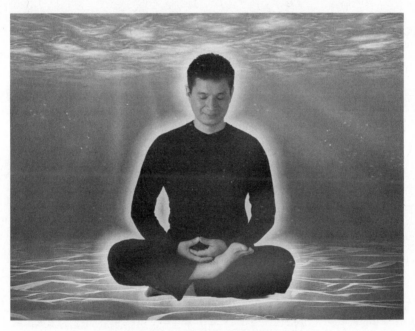

Figure 1.4: Sitting or lying in an ocean of Qi

1. Lie or sit down comfortably on your back, hands by your side.

2. Breathe naturally.

3. You are a sponge floating underwater in the ocean.

4. Light from above penetrates the water. It penetrates you.

5. The water is golden and bright.

6. You are soft and open.

7. The Qi of the Universe is penetrating every cell of your body.

8. *I am in Qi; Qi is in me.*

9. The ocean is endless and boundless. It extends to the ends of the Universe. You are endless and boundless.

10. Dissolve into this ocean. You are bright and light, endless and boundless.

11. Nourish your Qi until you are ready to open your eyes, feeling refreshed and energized.

Nourishing Qi is a practice that ends every exercise. This practice allows the energies you cultivate to settle down and rebalance naturally. The less you do while practicing, the more you experience a sense of deep relaxation. Falling asleep while practicing is a sign that deep healing may be taking place. Simply allow whatever arises to unfold naturally and without interference.

2

Mind as Number

The Mystery of Being

Twenty thousand years ago, a Paleolithic hunter is gazing up at the lights flickering in the sky on a chilly spring night. The shaman had a dream at the new moon. She said the woolly mammoth would return before the next full moon. "Go, watch for their arrival," she instructed the young men of the tribe. And on this night, the hunter and his kinsmen are perched on an outcrop overlooking the valley waiting for the rumbling. Listening to the silence, he is mesmerized by the shimmering stars. There are so many. They are so beautiful. His awareness melts into the vastness of space and for a few timeless breaths he is connected to all that is. Another hunter makes a sound that breaks the reverie, but the man is left pondering, Who am I? Who are you? Why does anything exist? What is going on? No answer is forthcoming. It is a mystery.

Three days pass before the romp of the mammoth herd unsettles the ground. At daybreak, the hunters are ready for them. Working as a tight-knit group they goad the mammoths with spears and shrieks and set their sight on a young bull. They surround him, close in cautiously, and attack fiercely. Spears protrude from the wounded beast. The hunter approaches the mammoth ready to cast his spear but the wild animal spins around and swipes its powerful trunk across his neck. The hunter falls unconscious as the mammoth rises on its hind legs and stomps him. The mammoth is speared by the other hunters and falls to the ground bleeding and whimpering beside the dead man.

The two dead bodies lie listless on the ground. The hunters form a circle around their fallen kinsman. A few moments ago, their brother was vital and full of life. Now, he lies motionless on the ground. A body without breath. Where is he? What is death? Another mystery.

The dead hunter's pregnant wife is in labor. Two moons have passed since she lost her mate. The female elders are chanting in her hut. The rest of the tribe is drumming outside. They are guiding in the spirit that will be born through her. The chanting and the drumming stops. An infant cry pierces the silence. A girl is born. The mother embraces her child. Holding the tiny, precious miracle, she marvels at her child and sheds tears of joy. The infant is nursing. Who is this being? What is life? Another mystery.

Two hundred centuries have passed. We are the progeny of the progeny of stone age tribes. We have accumulated mountains of knowledge. We know about atoms and can build cars. We know about tectonic plates and can build microchips. Knowledge continues to sprint at an accelerated rate. We are numerate and literate. We create computers and possess a universe of knowledge at our fingertips. More books exist than we could speed read in a thousand lifetimes. And yet, who hasn't looked up at the starry sky and wondered why the universe exists? We are taught that 13.8 billion years ago there was a Big Bang, and we are able to trace the history of the universe to within three minutes of its inception. But what prompted the Big Bang? The laws of science break down before that three-minute mark. Science cannot answer that question. The Big Bang was preceded by a big shrug. Knowledge crumbles at the foothills of Creation. No one knows why anything exists at all. The mystery of existence remains as mysterious as it was twenty thousand years ago.

Who hasn't lost a dear friend or close relative? We fall into the yawning abyss of chaos when we hear the news. When death breaks into our lives, we feel helpless. The hard edges of the everyday world crumble and we enter an otherworldly trance. Who hasn't crossed paths with death and wondered about their own mortality? One day, we will be the one who dies and news of our passing will open the gates of grief in the hearts of those who love us. The mystery of death remains unsolved.

Who hasn't held a delicate newborn infant and wondered about the miracle of life? How does matter draw on itself and become animate? How do minerals, liquids, and gases coalesce into sentient beings capable of playing poker? The mystery of life remains unsolved.

Despite all the impressive knowledge we have gathered, life, death, and existence itself remain an ever-present mystery. Our lives are bounded by these mysteries from beginning to end and every moment in between. We are known as homo sapiens sapiens, the humans who know that they know. And it is true that we know that we know. We possess the capacity to reflect on our knowledge. But the primordial mysteries of death, life, and existence transcend our knowledge.

Picture the tree of knowledge that grows a branch with every new discovery. It is easy to envision this majestic tree and miss the obvious. The roots that sustain the tree are invisible. Given the hardship and adversity of life, we sidestep the unknowable aspects of our being. We have bills to pay. The news cycle diverts our attention one way and then the other. We escape the heaviness of the daily grind through pleasure and entertainment. We suffer the wounds of love. We fight to protect. We focus on deadlines and goals; we jump between meetings and presentations. And in the hubbub of life, we ignore the primal questions until we occasionally meld into the mesmerizing sky and remember the mystery of our being, or encounter incipient life or mortality.

But some people are born to wonder about the mysteries. They cannot stop inquiring about the primal questions. They become fixated on the invisible roots. They become seekers of absolute and timeless truths and devote themselves to the exploration of the unknowable. Throughout the ages and across all cultures and traditions, these mystical explorers sought answers to the great mystery of being. These men and women drew on the spiritual traditions to explore otherworldly realities. Through long periods of fasting and meditation, and by entering into altered states of consciousness, some of them realized the unknowable and returned from their inner sojourns with ecstatic pearls of wisdom.

The sages of the wisdom traditions invariably teach that the language that we use to describe concrete events in the mundane world is inadequate to the task of describing transcendent truths. The first verse of the Dao De Jing reads, *The Dao that can be named is not the absolute Dao*. Plato's *Allegory of the Cave* offers a similar vision. How can a person who lives in a cave their entire life staring at shadows on the wall understand the glow and radiance of the sun? God in the Bible is famously invisible, unknowable, and nameless.

Sages agree: The ultimate mystery cannot be reduced to words or understood intellectually. But the ultimate mystery *can* be experienced. You can awaken and realize your true nature, and once you do, everything you knew about reality changes. Mystics teach that when you awaken to true nature you become immortal, you merge with God, you become One with all things, you ascend to Heaven, you attain Nirvana, you dissolve into the Supreme Ultimate, you extinguish your identity, you reunite with the Dao. The words are powerful words but they are still words. You can read the last sentence over and over, memorize it and recite it in sixty-seven languages three times a day, but that knowledge won't get you any closer to the truth than eating a laminated menu will satisfy your hunger.

The way to pierce through the veil of the mysteries and experience of your authentic nature is by undertaking a journey to Spirit. In the age of airplanes and cars, a journey often means flying a jet across the tallest mountains and the deepest seas for a few hours before landing, staying in a comfortable hotel, and taking bus tours of the local tourist sites and museums. But think back to a time when a journey involved months of preparation and years of exploration through unknown lands. There were wild animals, extreme weather, and bandits to fend off. If you ever reached your destination, you would return transformed. You would be wiser and bring back stories that would bewilder and amaze those who never left their homes.

A spiritual journey is more like a traditional adventure requiring serious preparation and a long-term commitment. In fact, we are all on a spiritual journey, whether we realize it or not. It is a voyage that began at birth and ends at death. It is a journey bordered by two of the great mysteries. And in between those two points, our spiritual journey is cradled by the mystery of our existence.

Life begins with an inhale and ends with an exhale, and all day long we breathe in and breathe out. Every mindful breath is a recollection of the primal questions. Mindful breathing is the simplest way to engage the spiritual journey mindfully. With your next inhale, become mindful of the long chain of inhalations leading to your first in-breath, and with your next exhale, become mindful of the chain of exhalations that lead to your final out-breath. And in the pause between inhale and exhale, become mindful of the moment of stillness that represents the mystery of your being. Life, death, and your being are encapsulated in every breath that you take. Every breath is a silent inquiry into the primal questions. Mindful breathing is a simple yet profound meditation practice that embraces the ineffable mysteries of life, death, and existence.

Exercise 4: Mindful Breathing

1. Adopt Natural Sitting Posture (Exercise 1).

2. Inhale and become aware of your birth.

3. At the pause between breaths, become aware of the mystery of your being.

4. Exhale and become aware of your mortality.

5. Become aware of the mysteries that your existence embodies. Awaken the remarkable fact of your existence. *I exist!*

6. Repeat nine times or more.

7. Nourish your Qi (Exercise 3). *I am in Qi; Qi is in me.*

From One to Zero

Despite the nebulous mysteries toward which spirituality orients, the meditations that lead to the realization of those mysteries is rigorously scientific in nature. A spiritual master imparts meditation instructions to a student who practices the exercises precisely, and the anticipated results are achieved. Another student practices and the results are validated once again. The predicted outcome of meditation practice has been corroborated by thousands of practitioners over the course of centuries. The difference between natural science and spiritual science is that spiritual science is validated through inner experience. The spiritual journey is a scientific process that unfolds inwardly. Xiao Yao learned meditation practices from his teacher and I am imparting these practices to you. They worked for him, they worked for me, and they will work for you.

Although Xiao Yao was a Buddhist monk, his teachings incorporated many Daoist meditations. Our spiritual journey follows a Daoist path flavored with Buddhist insights into the nature of mind. We begin that journey by establishing a philosophical map of the territory that we will traverse experientially in later chapters. This map extends from One to Two, from Two to Three, from Three to Ten Thousand, and from Ten Thousand to Zero. Each of these numbers symbolizes a cosmological principle that is embodied by an aspect of the human mind.

One: Wuji

Dao gives birth to One.

Dao De Jing, Chapter 42[1]

In Daoist philosophy, the name given to the realm of Oneness is Wuji (woo-jee). Wuji means having no opposition, duality, or polarity. This is a realm where difference, contradiction, opposition, hypocrisy, antagonism, dissent, argumentation, division, competition, strife, conflict, or fragmentation of any sort do not exist. Wuji is the unified realm of Perfect Peace. Wuji is the undifferentiated bedrock of awareness from which the countless expressions of duality arise.

All form arises from Wuji. Your values, your big toe, the pizza you ate last night and are still digesting, the itch you just scratched— every sensory experience arises from Wuji. Any rational and irrational thought that arises in awareness, arises from Wuji. And yet, Wuji is

---

1   All quotes from the Dao De Jing are translated interpretations by the authors.

imperceptible like the roots of the tree of knowledge. It is ungraspable by the senses or their technological extensions. Wuji cannot be touched, or seen, or heard. Picture a movie screen. One day, the screen portrays a love story that brings the audience to tears. Another day, a thriller has the audience on the edge of their seat. Another day a horror movie has the audience squirming and screaming. The movie screen does not change each time the theater shows a new film. The screen is perfectly unified and featureless. It is imperceptible and goes unnoticed while the images flow and the stories drag us along. And yet without the screen, those stories would scatter into incoherent light.

At the human level, Wuji can be envisioned as the blank screen of awareness on which our lives are projected. Everything arising in consciousness arises on the screen of Wuji. The fragrance of the most delicate flower arises on the screen of Wuji. The thrill of a first date and your heart-felt prayers for a dear friend in need arise on the screen of Wuji. Everything that is subject to change arises on the screen of Wuji. The unchanging and formless nature of the screen establishes Wuji as an absolute feature of our being. It is the steady anchor of ever-changing consciousness.

The realm of Wuji is perfectly unified. Imagine attending a concert where a beloved song is performed in a large hall by a cherished performer. The crowd bursts into spontaneous song at the refrain. You find yourself singing along with everyone else. A deep sense of peacefulness unites the listeners. The audience is swaying in unison to the melody, and everyone feels connected to everyone else. That feeling of union captures the nature of Wuji. Imagine that you are in the presence of a spiritual master in a serene temple setting. Your eyes are closed, and you are absorbed in peaceful silence. You lose your ordinary sense of time and drift into an altered state of perfect stillness. Your mind is perfectly still. Your heart is perfectly still. Your body is perfectly still. That perfect stillness negates thoughts, feeling, and sensations. Mental activity, emotional activity, and physical activity are wholly absent. There are no objects and no subjects to divide attention. The union that arises at the concert and the stillness generated by the meditation hints at the perfection that arises when the mind abides in Wuji.

The word we assign the aspect of mind that is still, unified, and perfectly peaceful is *Spirit*. Spirit is Wuji personified. Spirit is the mind at peace. Wuji is the abode of Spirit. Most of our minds are detached from Spirit. We suffer from amnesia. The coconut has fallen from the tree of life and bonked our head. We have forgotten about our fundamental nature as Spirit. Our minds are endlessly divided. Yet every night, our mind reverts to Wuji when we fall asleep and surrender our ordinary waking awareness and enter the realm of deep, dreamless sleep. If you were able to awaken awareness during deep, dreamless sleep, you would realize the perfection of Wuji and your nature as Spirit.

Recall the feeling of well-being that accompanies a deeply satisfying night of sleep. The moment that you wake up, you still experience a tinge of sublime peacefulness and serenity. Those are the trailing clouds of spiritual glory that emanate from Wuji. Now imagine that you can enter the realm of Wuji consciously and experience the sublime peace of Spirit while awake and fully conscious. Your mind would be alert and perfectly still. There would be no thought. There would be no objects or subjects, no duality, no mental chatter. No division. No confusion. No emotions. No desires. Just the Perfect Peace and stillness of unified oneness as you perceive the world around you.

Through meditation practice, you can learn to awaken Wuji and abide as Spirit at will. There is a passageway within your body that enables your awareness to enter the realm of Wuji. Once that portal is open, you can enter Wuji at will, abide as Spirit, and experience Perfect Peace consciously. And when you end your meditation, you can keep the connection between Spirit and the ordinary world.

An encounter between our ordinary mind and unified mind, Spirit, can arise spontaneously, during moments of sincere prayer or when we are involved in a creative endeavor. The "eureka" moment, when an original vision is conceived, represents the union of everyday mind with Spirit. During a creative moment, Spirit embraces the ordinary mind. We disappear for an instant, and when we reemerge, we experience an expansion of consciousness, a lightness of being, and an original vision. Imagine a writer with a creative block. She closes her eyes and her mind reaches down the well of creativity from which she draws inspiration. She disappears for a timeless moment and returns from the experience with a novel vision that inspires her work. The inspiration of creativity emanates from Wuji.

Each one of us is working on a story—the story of our life—which is shaped by the degree of creativity that we are able to channel into the choices that we make. The more intimate you become with Wuji, the more meaningful your worldly life becomes. When you abide as Spirit, the realm of Oneness becomes your home. Life becomes a blessing. Once you identify as Spirit—once you step out into the world of duality and radiate the quality of Perfect Peace—you become a blessing in the lives of others.

In Daoist philosophy, Wuji, Spirit, and Perfect Peace are symbolized by the blank circle shown in Figure 2.1 below.

Figure 2.1: Empty Circle

Two and Three: Greater Duality and Lesser Duality (Yin and Yang)

One gives birth to Two.
Two gives birth to Three.
Dao De Jing, Chapter 42

From the oneness of Wuji, the mind enters the realm of duality. At the level of Spirit, there is only one item on the menu: perfection. Once we enter the realm of duality, we leave perfection behind and a new quality emerges: free will. At the heart of duality resides the mind's ability to choose. And the quality of those choices determines the quality of our lives. Daoist sages divided duality into two aspects, Greater Duality and Lesser Duality, or Liang Yi and Si Xiang in Chinese.

Greater Duality—Greater Duality is the aspect of duality that emerges from One and is associated with the number Two. Imagine drawing a line down the middle of the circle of Wuji and dividing oneness in half. See Figure 2.2 below.

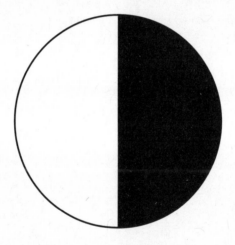

Figure 2.2: Half Circle

The divided circle symbolizes Greater Duality and the free will it engenders. The two sides of the circle represent the most fundamental choice that confronts free will: the choice between good and evil. We are free to choose good and we are free to choose evil. Nothing stands in the way of free will and the choice that we make shapes the reality we create for ourselves.

Epic stories such as *Star Wars*, *Harry Potter*, *Game of Thrones*, and *The Lord of the Rings* base their plotlines on the struggle between good and evil.

In each instance, protagonists must make a choice. It is not an easy choice to make. Evil is glamorous, tempting, and seductive. It promises power, fortune, and fame. Does the hero succumb to evil or step into the heroic spotlight and struggle against evil in the name of goodness? The epic stories that capture the collective imagination of entire generations are cautionary tales about the eternal battle between these two irreconcilable sides. Contemporary epic stories are a retelling of the same struggle told by ancient cultures. Stories of Bronze Age heroes battling monsters, Iron Age forces of light battling forces of darkness, and medieval angels battling demons are the same stories retold in different historical contexts. The epic battle between good and evil was relevant centuries ago and continues to be relevant today because this struggle is not just the struggle of imaginary heroes, but it is our struggle as well.

When our mind awakens Greater Duality, we stand at a crossroads and our free will has to choose between following the high road and following the low road. The high road is the path that we follow when we are guided by benevolence. The low road is the path that we follow when we are guided by malevolence. The latter leads to catastrophe, destruction, and doom.

One woman dives into turbulent waters to save a child from drowning. Another traffics vulnerable children for profit. The line between good and evil is bipartisan. We don't need a university degree to distinguish good from evil. We recognize good and evil universally. Betraying a friend is never a good thing. Violating trust for personal gain is never a good thing. Incriminating the innocent is never a good thing. When something is never good, it is evil by definition. Protecting the vulnerable is always a good thing. Helping the helpless is always a good thing. Healing the sick is always a good thing. And when something is never evil, it is good by definition.

The eternal truth that arises at the level of Greater Duality is that good and evil are universal forces. It is a timeless struggle that each one of us must wage. When a choice at the level of Greater Duality needs to be made, there is no room for compromise. That choice is definitive. When the mind is poised to make a choice between good and evil, our conscience is awakened. Conscience is the voice of free will that steers us toward good. The stronger our conscience, the easier it is to choose good. As our conscience weakens, we are more likely to incline toward evil. Once we choose evil, if we still possess conscience, we experience guilt. If we lack the capacity for feeling any remorse for our malevolence—if we lack a conscience—we become an expression of pure evil. Pure evil revels in destruction, horror, and hate. A mind abiding in that state is the enemy of humanity.

When conscience steers us toward good, we feel gratitude, grace, and blessed. When we feel that we have no choice but to choose good over evil, we become pure good. Pure good revels in virtue and the love of humanity. The choice between good and evil is a choice between love and hate and you are free to choose as you will.

Life presents us with ample opportunities to choose between good and evil and to exercise our free will on a daily basis. Should I betray a co-worker to advance my position? Should I violate trust to enrich myself? Should I demonize another to make myself more appealing? Should I pray for the destruction of another human being? A cruel leader who uses malice to advance a personal agenda is serving evil. A corrupt judge that takes the bribe and sentences the innocent is evil. A rumor monger who spreads a falsehood to get ahead is evil. The temptation of evil is an ever-present lure on the spiritual path. Buddha and Jesus both had to contend with the temptation of evil on their way to liberation and salvation. As we advance on the spiritual journey, it is essential that we remain vigilant and choose the high road. The eternal truth teaches us to unequivocally embrace benevolence and the love of humanity and to reject malevolence, which tempts us through the promise of power, riches, and fame.

Spiritual seekers often spend years purifying themselves in preparation for their awakening as Spirit. A conscience free of guilt and a benevolent mind are the key to entering Wuji. The road to perfection passes through the land of purity. If we are serious about abiding as Spirit and tasting perfection, we must embody good and attain Pure Mind. Pure Mind is the exalted expression of twoness just as Spirit is the exalted expression of oneness.

Lesser Duality—Lesser Duality, Si Xiang, is associated with the number Three. After the oneness of Spirit and the twoness of Pure Mind, we encounter the three-ness of Higher Mind. At the level of Pure Mind, the choice between good and evil is clear-cut. Brutalizing an old woman to finance a drug habit is *never* a good choice to make. Torturing a pet for fun is *never* a good choice. Planting evidence to falsely convict the innocent is *never* a good choice to make. Choices made at the level of Pure Mind are universally self-evident.

But not all choices are self-evident. Is it right to be conservative or is it right to be liberal? Is it right to be strict or is it right to be lenient? What is the right choice: liberty or equality? In answering these last questions, did you identify with one set of answers over another? And if you met an individual who chose the opposite answers, would you be able to get along with that person? Or would you polarize and repel each other like magnets?

While the distinctions made at the level of Greater Duality are bipartisan, the choices made at the level of Lesser Duality are partisan and often polarize the mind. While the choice between good and evil is eternally true, the choice between right and wrong is relatively true. Sometimes liberty is right and sometimes liberty is wrong. Sometimes equality is right and sometimes equality is wrong. The opposite of a relative truth is another relative truth. Think of it this way: Breathing is always good. Wearing a sweater can be the right thing to do or the wrong thing to do depending on the weather. The relative truths of Lesser Duality depend on the broader context and are subject to debate.

Relative truths are not "absolutely" good or evil and treating them as such results in polarization and tension. I am pointing a finger at you while you are pointing a finger at me. I can't prove you wrong and I can't prove to you that I'm right. And neither can you. I am convinced that I am right and you are wrong. You are convinced that I am wrong and that you are right. *Always conservative! Always liberal! Always freedom! Always equality!* A polarized mind privileges one relative truth and seeks supremacy, power, and domination over the other relative truth, and when that happens, strife becomes a way of life and conflict ensues.

Arguments between relative truths can never be absolutely won by either side because both sides of a polarity are partially right and partially wrong. Liberty and equality are both right and wrong. Too much liberty leads to imbalance. Too much conformity leads to imbalance as well. Too many rules lead to disharmony. Too few rules lead to disharmony as well. Depending on the context, one relative truth may be appropriate, and its polar opposite be appropriate in another context.

The role of Higher Mind is to recognize the antagonism between two relative truths, and to integrate the polarities by invoking a higher principle. For example, the higher principle that integrates liberty and equality is fairness. Sometimes fairness leans toward liberty and sometimes toward equality. When two individuals with opposing views related to this polarity awaken Higher Mind, their dialogue will converge on a resolution that centers on fairness and resolves the tension. When two individuals with opposing views related to this polarity do not awaken Higher Mind, a sense of injustice prevails that will drive a never-ending cycle of conflict and retribution. Higher principles include fairness, care, courage, responsibility, and honesty, among others. The fundamental point to recall about Higher Mind is that *any* polarity can be integrated by invoking the *right* higher principle.

Each instance of Lesser Duality includes two relative truths and a higher principle that holds the key to integrating that polarity. For this reason, the number three, which symbolizes stability, balance, and harmony, is associated with Higher Mind. Higher principles bind together to create moral codes intended to preserve balance and harmony within society. Unlike eternal codes of good and evil that remain unchanging, moral codes shift over time like desert sands. These shifts are natural and necessary as societies adapt to changing life conditions. What was deemed moral just one generation ago may be deemed immoral today. Higher Mind is the aspect of mind that mediates between those divergent points of view to bring about harmony through moral reasoning. While Pure Mind relates to the free will and the choice between good and evil, Higher Mind relates to moral principles that bring about harmony and balance.

Each one of us can reach for the right moral principal when the need arises to right a perceived wrong and bring about accord. An employer that has cultivated Higher Mind is able to preserve harmony and balance in the workspace by invoking the principle of respect. A politician that has cultivated Higher Mind is able to preserve harmony and balance in society by invoking the principle of responsibility. A parent that has cultivated Higher Mind is able to preserve harmony and balance in the family through the principle of care.

The Daoist sages who mapped out the spiritual path symbolized the concept of Higher Mind and relative truth by morphing the straight line dividing the circle of Greater Duality into the swerving line of Lesser Duality. See Figure 2.3 below.

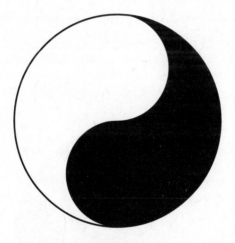

Figure 2.3: Yin Yang No Dots

The straight line dividing the circle of Greater Duality represents Pure Mind, eternal truth, and good and evil, while the swerving line dividing the circle of Lesser Duality represents Higher Mind, relative truth, polarities, and higher principles. The straight line of Greater Duality can be thought of as the far side of the moon, which always faces away from the earth. Likewise, eternal truths are perpetual and unchanging. The swerving line of Lesser Duality can be envisioned as the ever-changing play of light and shadow on a hill over the course of the day.

Picture a hill with the sun shining directly overhead. It is noontime. The entire hill is bathed in glorious light. There are no shadows to be seen anywhere. As the sun moves past the zenith and begins its descent, budding shadows emerge and lengthen as afternoon progresses. As sunset approaches, half the hill is submerged in darkness and the other is glowing in twilight. As evening sets in, shadows overtake both sides of the hill, and as the faint hues of day fade away, darkness overtakes the hill. At midnight, the starry sky can be seen above while the hill below is draped in darkness. After midnight, the nighttime sky gradually lightens until sunrise unbinds the hold of darkness. A point of light breaks over the horizon at dawn and light spreads over one half of the hill as morning surges and another day begins.

If you observed the interplay of light and shadow on that hill over a twenty-four-hour period with a time-lapse camera, you would witness the interplay of light and shadow as depicted in Figure 2.4 below.

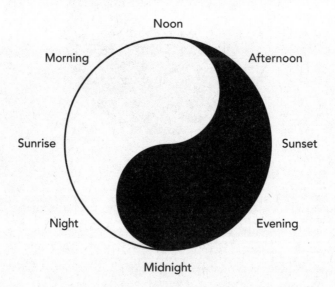

Figure 2.4: Yin Yang Times of Day

The Chinese name for the light side of a hill is Yang and the name of the shadowy side of the hill is Yin. From the perspective of Greater duality, Yang implies *always good* while Yin implies *always evil*. Topping a pizza with deadly mushrooms is never a good idea. It is absolute Yin. A lifesaving antidote, on the other hand, is always good. It is absolute Yang. From the perspective of Lesser Duality, however, both Yin and Yang are right and wrong. Is morning better than evening? Is sunset right and sunrise wrong? Daoist sages viewed the Yin and Yang of Lesser Duality as equally good, equally powerful, and equally necessary to achieve and maintain balance and harmony. Can relative Yin exist without relative Yang? Can left exist without right? Can up exist without down? At the level of Higher Mind, Yin and Yang continuously dance around each other to restore harmony. The swerving shape between them represents the intelligence of Higher Mind that preserves the balance that arises when polarities are properly integrated.

Multiplicity: The Ten Thousand Things

The Three birth the Ten Thousand Things.

Dao De Jing, Chapter 42

An observant person would point out that day and night are not equal. The daily cycle unfolds within the yearly cycle. In the spring and summer, days are longer, and the hill reflects more light over the course of a given twenty-four-hour period. In the fall and winter, darkness covers the hill for a longer stretch of time. Collectively, daytime in the summer is relatively more Yang, while wintertime and nighttime is relatively more Yin than at other times of the year. To further complicate the situation, the moon also undergoes transformations of light and shadow throughout the month. The full moon represents the time of maximum Yang in the lunation cycle while the new moon is the time of maximum Yin.

A full moon in winter at noon represents Yang and Yin and Yang. A new moon in summer at midnight represents Yin and Yang and Yin. The circadian, diurnal, and lunation cycles unfold in relationship to each other so that in practice Yin unfolds within Yang and Yang unfolds within Yin. The relationship between Yin and Yang becomes immensely complicated as we investigate the nature of duality in the context of the physical world that we experience through our senses.

At the level of Greater Duality, the distinction between Yin and Yang is clear-cut and easy to discern: good versus evil. At the level of Lesser Duality, the distinction between Yin and Yang becomes rational, dialectical, and relativistic. But when Daoist sages considered the nature of duality in the everyday world, they were confronted with a high degree of complexity. The number of iterations of Yin and Yang required to describe the changes unfolding in the material world increased exponentially. Daoist sages developed systems such as the Yi Jing that distinguishes sixty-four different combinations of Yin and Yang using hexagrams. It would have been impractical to extend that system into a more elaborate structure that involved hundreds, thousands, or millions of iterations, so they stopped at sixty-four.

The Daoist sages intuited that Yin and Yang ultimately described the structure of the material world, but they lacked the scientific tools to validate their theory. They did not know about subatomic particles, atoms, molecules, and cells. They did not know about the four fundamental forces of nature. They lacked the technological means to extend their senses beyond the bounds of human perception. And yet, from what they were able to observe, they presumed that the world of material form is made up of countless iterations of Yin and Yang. Technically, they were right and modern science has come to the same conclusion.

A simple way to grasp the idea that the world is made of Yin and Yang is to consider the digital world created by a computer game. At the machine language level, countless strings made up of zeros and ones organize the rules of play and create the images and sounds that drive the action. The gamer who is yelping excitedly at the screen does not perceive those zeros and ones, just a space laser zapping an endless stream of snarling aliens. Modern science describes the dynamics of physics, chemistry, and biology in terms of attraction and repulsion. Positively charged atoms are attracted to negatively charged atoms. Positively charged atoms are repelled by other positively charged atoms. Negatively charged atoms are repelled by other negatively charged atoms. The Yin and Yang of attraction and repulsion form the binary strings of zeros and ones that organize the laws of physics, chemistry, and biology that create the multiplicity of forms that we perceive through our physical senses.

The atoms that make up the molecules, that make up the cells, that make up your body are held together by the power of attraction. Your body is attracted to the earth by gravity. The earth is attracted to the sun. The moon is attracted to the earth and to the sun. The sun is attracted to the galactic center. Attraction holds the Universe together and repulsion sets it in motion. Up and down the orders of magnitude that define the observable Universe, we encounter Yin and Yang in action.

When the human senses interact with the physical world, Practical Mind arises. Practical Mind is the aspect of mind that likes and dislikes. It is attracted and repulsed and reacts accordingly. I like spicy food and you dislike spicy food. Spicy food is not good or evil. Spicy food is not right or wrong. It can be liked or disliked by anyone with impunity. Practical Mind is attracted to some things and repelled by others. I like action films. I like tennis. I like reading ancient mystical texts. I like the sound of a gurgling stream. I like roller coasters. I am drawn toward all of those things. And maybe you dislike all of the things that I like. And that's fine.

At the level of Spirit, we all like the same perfection and there is nothing to dislike. At the level of Pure Mind, we all like good and we all dislike evil. At the level of Higher Mind, both polarities are partly right and partly wrong—we like and dislike them both simultaneously. At the level of Practical Mind, we each like what we like and we each dislike what we dislike.

Practical Mind is attracted to activities that it likes, and it becomes increasingly proficient at those activities. The activities that we like most define our identity in the world. Someone who likes playing with children is more likely to become a daycare teacher. Someone who likes performing in public is more likely to become an actor. Someone who likes cooking is more likely to become a chef. The more skilled we become at something that we like, the more likely we are to attract people who can benefit from our expertise. If you need help fixing a leaky faucet, you call a plumber. If you have a problem with your foot, a podiatrist can help. If your car breaks down, a mechanic can fix it. At its best, Practical Mind likes to fix problems and service needs. Practical Mind is the skilled and expert mind of an individual. Collectively, the Practical Minds of the members of a community enable the smooth functioning of that society. When Practical Mind is not pursuing its likes, we feel broken and fragmented. We feel disconnected from the mainstream. We feel lonely. We feel useless and the world becomes a desolate place.

Practical Mind is guided toward proficiency by following objective truth. Let's say you want to bake cookies and you read online that soft cookies require 375 degrees for twelve to fifteen minutes, and if you want crispy cookies, bake them at 425 degrees between eight to ten minutes. Those statements are both objectively true in the world of cookies. You can verify them for yourself with a few ingredients. If you read on another site that you should bake cookies for six hours at 500 degrees and followed those instructions, you would end up with inedible charred cookies. That recipe is a falsehood, and it would be quickly discarded for being untrue.

Objective truth is a factual truth on which we can all agree. You step on a scale and the readout shows a number. You can't argue with that number. That number is not good or evil. It is not right or wrong. Any scale on the planet that is functioning properly will display the correct weight. If a scale contradicted that number, it would be incorrect. Any deviation from objective truth is a falsehood. The way to succeed in the empirical world is by following factual knowledge that derives from the objective truth. Incorrect knowledge leads to abject failure.

Daoist sages referred to the immensity of the physical world as the Ten Thousand Things. Why Ten Thousand? If you had to count a thousand apples, it would take you a while. If you finally reached a thousand apples and were told that you had to count another nine thousand, you would probably recoil at the task. Ten Thousand is a catchall phrase that means more than you care to count. The sages symbolized the Ten Thousand Things by adding two dots on the swirls of Yin and Yang depicted in Figure 2.5. The dots represent the manifest world. They represent Yin within Yang and Yang within Yin ad infinitum. They represent the fractal tree of attraction and repulsion that holds the Universe together. They represent Practical Mind and objective truth. They represent empirical knowledge. They represent your likes and dislikes. They represent your technical expertise. The represent the factual knowledge required to bake two cookies, one soft and the other one crispy.

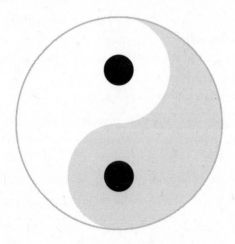

Figure 2.5: The Dots Emerge

Zero: Dao

Dao gives birth to One
One gives birth to Two
Two gives birth to Three
Three gives birth to the Ten Thousand Things
The Ten Thousand Things yield to Yin and embrace Yang.

Dao De Jing, Chapter 42

We leave Dao for last because it is first. And it is first, but it is not One. But it is also One. It is not One and it is One. Both are true. The paradoxical nature of these statements reflects the paradoxical nature of Dao.

We cannot begin to make sense of Dao until we grasp One, Two, Three, and Ten Thousand. And despite our attempt at making sense of Dao, nothing we say about Dao truly makes sense.

We are calling Dao "Dao" rather than "The Dao" because Dao is not an object out there that we can point to like "the chair." It is not a subject that we hold in our minds either like, "the feeling of joy." Dao abides invisibly at the center of every object and every subject. It is everywhere and nowhere. It is always and never. It is fullness and emptiness. It is being and nonbeing. It is all of these contrasts manifesting simultaneously across all the realms of existence and nonexistence.

Dao precedes One in the way that zero precedes the number one. One is something. Dao is nothing. And yet Dao is also everything. Dao is the Daoist equivalent of God in theistic religion. The aspects of mind that arise at One, Two, Three, and Ten Thousand each conceptualize Dao in partial and limited ways. Spirit envisions Dao as perfect. But Spirit, perfectly unified and at peace, cannot grasp the paradoxical nature of Dao. Dao cannot be reduced to perfection because it includes the imperfections inherent in duality. Pure Mind envisions Dao as good. And yet Dao transcends good because it allows evil to exist. Higher Mind envisions Dao in terms of higher principles such as care, justice, and nobility. And yet Dao also includes polarity, imbalance, and disharmony. Practical Mind negates Dao since it is imperceptible and irreducible to time, matter, or energy, and yet Dao is that unknowable nothing that enables everything the senses grasp to arise.

Dao is the sheath of nonbeing that enfolds all that is. Dao implies the nothing that enfolds everything and the never that enfolds always. Dao swaddles perfect and imperfect, good and evil, right and wrong, true and false. Like the number zero, it cannot be divided or multiplied. It is neither big nor small. Dao is Zero. Dao is the void in which everything arises, all things abide, and to which everything returns. Dao is the nothing at the heart of all things.

Dao is symbolized by the same image that we encounter in Figure 2.5, but it is interpreted differently.

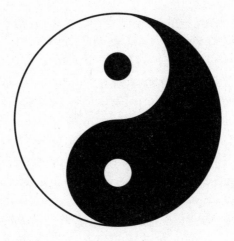

Figure 2.6: Taiji

While Figure 2.5 emphasizes the two dots representing the Ten Thousand Things, Figure 2.5 symbolizes the wholeness of Dao, which includes Wuji, Greater and Lesser Yin and Yang, and the Ten Thousand Things. The way to interpret Figure 2.6 from the perspective of Dao is to awaken the meaning of the unified circle, the two swirls, and the two dots, and to recognize that all the realms of reality and all the aspects of mind are expressions of Dao. Ultimately, all arises from emptiness, being arises from nonbeing, and everything arises from nothing. Dao adds nothing to the symbol and yet it changes everything about it.

The symbol of Dao is known as Taiji, the Supreme Ultimate. Taiji symbolizes the essence of Daoism. If you grasp the principles enshrined in Taiji, you grasp the philosophy of Daoism. If you embody the principles enshrined in Taiji, you attain immortality. By awakening Taiji, we become aware of Zero. We awaken the emptiness of Dao—the nonbeing that sustains our being. We create space in awareness for the nothing that is everything. Taiji is a powerful symbol that opens the door of the mind to the Supreme Ultimate.

While there is nothing that we can say directly about Dao, we can dance around Dao and tease out a few paradoxical insights about the void in all things. A question we can ask about Dao is, Why did Dao not stop at the perfection of One? Why manifest duality and multiplicity? Why didn't emptiness simply create Spirit and abide in Perfect Peace eternally? Why create imperfection? Why create desire and suffering? The closest that we can come to offering a coherent answer to these questions rests with the following paradoxical thought: perfection is imperfect and imperfection enables perfection to become more perfect. Imagine that you are perfectly at peace floating around in a heavenly cloud. Would you ever want to leave your cloud? Would you ever learn to crawl or walk? Would you learn how to read and write? Would you ever get up to go to work? Would you ever do anything? Would anything or anyone ever develop or grow? The answer is no. Why leave your heavenly cloud if you can abide in perfection forever? Perfection is imperfect because it fosters inertia. It lacks movement and growth. Imperfection creates possibilities. Imperfection presents the opportunity to evolve. Imperfection perfects perfection.

Another question: How does Dao motivate Spirit to enter duality? Dao spurs Spirit by doing nothing. Dao extends itself as the void and creates the empty space in which new possibilities can emerge. The nothing of Dao precipitates Spirit into duality. The emptiness of Dao awakens the sense of destiny. Destiny is a vacuum. Destiny is a void. Destiny is empty. Destiny is Zero. There is nothing there and yet this nothingness is the force that draws Spirit from the cloud of perfection out into the world. The draw of destiny is the emptiness that creates fullness. The draw of destiny is the nothingness that creates everything. The draw of destiny is the void of potential that engenders actualization. The draw of destiny creates time and space so that something can arise out of nothing. Destiny is the womb that conceives possibilities. The sense of emptiness, nothingness, and void that opens possibilities around time and space is the impetus that draws Spirit into manifestation. And since all things develop and evolve out of nothing, Dao is omniscient and omnipresent. Dao is the formless ground from which all forms emerge and to which they return. To awaken Dao is to realize that everything arises from emptiness, everything abides in emptiness, everything returns to emptiness. Everything arises from

Dao, everything abides in Dao, everything returns to Dao. Dao is nothing, and yet, Dao is everything, everywhere, and always.

In the human mind, Dao manifests as the sense of possibility that defines our personal destiny. Dao creates a void in our life that needs to be filled. Dao is the vacuum that spurs our Spirit into action. Dao arouses our Spirit with a sense of personal destiny. Dao generates a vision of idealized perfection that does not yet exist, and that vision inspires our Spirit and sets it in motion. As Spirit refracts into Pure Mind, the sense of good drives our sense of destiny toward realization. As Pure Mind refracts as Higher Mind, the sense of right drives our sense of destiny toward realization. As Higher Mind refracts into Practical Mind, the desire arises to master the practical skills required to actualize our destiny in the world. Through the outpouring of emptiness across the aspects of mind, the formless Dao manifests all form.

Perhaps Dao touches your Spirit with the feeling that it is your destiny to become a ballet dancer. You are not a ballet dancer in this moment, but you feel uplifted by the idea, and you envision yourself dancing on stage perfectly. You experience a sense of profound peace as you contemplate the vision. The desire to be good at ballet fills you with a deep sense of benevolence. You take classes and learn to embody balance and harmony through your movements. You practice until you perfect the skill. You become a proficient ballet dancer, and one day, while you are performing, your flawless dance fills the dance hall with a sense of perfect peace. Your Spirit is dancing on stage. You embody perfection and that perfection awakens a sense of profound peace in the audience. By offering your perfection to an imperfect world, you are realizing your destiny. As you bow on stage at the standing ovation, the wholeness of your being is bowing in gratitude. One, Two, Three, Ten Thousand, and Zero are all bowing. In that timeless moment, when the spotlight of existence honors your achievement, the meaning of your life is revealed.

The Chinese character for Dao means, *The Way*. The way to where? The way to a meaningful destination. For one person, The Way of Soccer may define their personal Dao. For another, the Dao of Accounting. Or the Dao of Parenting. Or the Dao of Engineering. Or the Dao of

Teaching. Once Dao touches our Spirit, we are going to experience meaning in the process of actualizing perfection. When we are walking the path of destiny, we are filled with a sense of purpose and our life makes sense.

Dao may touch our Spirit many times over the course of a single lifetime. Our sense of destiny can guide our career, relationships, education, friendships, and business prospects. Dao manifests mysteriously and sets our Spirit in motion in unique patterns of destiny that define the meaningful paths in our lives. As we pursue those meaningful paths, we grow by bringing our goodness to the world.

Our personal destinies are as unique as our fingerprints and stretch our lives in unique directions. But all human beings share one destiny in common, Great Dao. You may be a soccer star, an accounting wizard, a wonderful parent, a brilliant engineer, or a beloved teacher. Whatever personal Dao you are pursuing in the world, Great Dao is an invitation to every Spirit to awaken as Dao. Great Dao is the urge of awakened Spirit to awaken as the stillness of emptiness. Great Dao is the urge of Spirit to reunite with Dao. Great Dao is the urge of form to realize formlessness. Great Dao is the urge of One to merge into Zero.

Once Spirit awakens as Dao, we embody Great Dao. A spiritual master that awakens Great Dao abides as perfection in the world without having to do anything. There is no need to be a ballet dancer on stage to fill the audience hall with perfect peace. When Spirit reunites with Dao, perfection is no longer bound to a particular path, destiny, or vision. Dao is the emptiness that envelops everything, and when Spirit yields to Dao, perfection manifests everywhere, always. Perfection can wander into an elevator and speak to you. Perfection can drive a taxi. Perfection abiding as emptiness manifests effortlessly as it encounters the imperfections of the world. Great Dao is the eye of the hurricane that is perfectly still while all around the winds howl and the waves crash.

In Western terms, we can equate Dao with God and destiny with the will of God. When Spirit reunites with Dao—when Spirit merges with God—we become godly beings. We become divine and our divinity extends to all sentient beings. The suffering of all beings becomes our suffering. The sacrifices of a saint who has merged with God, the compassion of a Boddhisatva who has dissolved into Nirvana, the virtue of an Immortal that has reunited with Dao—these are all expressions of the same phenomenon.

The Vedic sages teach that only Brahma, Supreme God, is real and that the world is illusion. And yet they also teach that Brahma is the world. The Heart Sutra famously states that form is emptiness and emptiness is form. A Latin booklet written by an anonymous author defines God as an infinite sphere whose origin is everywhere and circumference is nowhere. Each of these paradoxical teachings affirms the non-dual or paradoxical nature of the Supreme Ultimate. Non-duality is the aspect of mind that has awakened Dao. Non-Dual Mind is the mind that perceives the One in the Many and the Many in the One. Non-Dual Mind perceives form as formless. Non-Dual Mind perceives the emptiness in fullness. Non-Dual Mind holds space for your reunion with Great Dao. Non-Dual Mind perceives you as an expression of Great Dao. The presence of a spiritual master prompts in the Spirit of a disciple the urge to awaken as Great Dao.

The spiritual journey is initiated by our sense of personal destiny. We strive to bring meaning into our lives by actualizing goodness, harmony and balance, and skillful expertise. We grow outwardly. And then we encounter a spiritual master and realize that the spiritual journey also leads inwardly toward Dao. We realize that perfection in the world is ephemeral and only covers a narrow band of experience. Our Spirit is touched by the awareness that we can embody perfection beyond space and time by reuniting with Dao. When our perfection abides in emptiness, we transcend time and space and realize Great Dao. This experience is the ultimate answer to the primal mysteries of life. A spiritual master who abides in Dao becomes immortal, transfigured, deified, holy. Reunion of Spirit with Dao completes the spiritual journey, although the spiritual journey never really ends since even a spiritual master has a personal destiny to fulfill by awakening the countless Spirits trapped in the world of form, suffering at the hands of evil, unaware that they are the children of Great Dao.

The table below summarizes the concepts we have covered.

Taiji	Realm	Truth	Perception	Awareness	Mind
Wuji	One	Absolute	Perfection	Unified and peaceful	Spirit
Greater Duality	Two	Eternal	Good and evil	Free will, conscience, and guilt	Pure Mind
Lesser Duality	Three	Relative	Right and wrong	Morals, principles, and reason	Higher Mind
Ten Thousand Things	Multiplicity	Objective	Correct and incorrect, like and dislike	Empirical knowledge and facts	Practical Mind
Dao	Void (Zero)	Paradoxical	Destiny, growth, and evolution	Emptiness and fullness	Non-dual Mind

Exercise 5: Taiji Breathing

Taiji is a symbol that we express with each breath. There are many kinds of breath: the breath of excitement, the breath of fear, the breath of sexual arousal, the breath of relaxation, the breath of laughter, the breath of serenity. The structure of all types of breath, however, is the same. We inhale, breathing pauses momentarily, we exhale, breathing pauses momentarily, and the cycle repeats. These four steps—inhale, pause, exhale, pause—are common to all breathing patterns. These four steps encapsulate the aspects of Taiji.

Inhalation represents Yin and embodies duality moving toward Spirit. The cessation of breath on the inhale is Wuji. Exhalation represents Yang and embodies duality moving toward matter. The pause of breath on the exhale is the Ten Thousand Things. Dao is implied by the emptiness of the lungs that creates the urge to inhale and the fullness of the lungs that creates the urge to exhale.

Taiji Breathing is a practice that transforms your breath into Taiji. We practice Taiji Breathing seated. We imagine that we are sitting at the center of a sphere that represents the Universe. That sphere can start off small and expand as we become more proficient at the practice. You inhale naturally through the nose, drawing in Qi from the surface of the sphere toward your Lower Dantian. You concentrate the Qi of the Universe at Lower Dantian as you complete the inhale. When your breathing pauses, become aware of your Lower Dantian. Lower Dantian is an energy point associated to Wuji. When your mind is centered on Lower Dantian, you are close to accessing Wuji. Allow your mind to rest at this point until the urge to breathe draws your exhale.

Exhale naturally through the nose radiating Qi from Lower Dantian in all directions to the edge of the sphere. Feel your Qi fill the universal sphere like air blown into a balloon. When the breath pauses, become aware of the sphere that represents the Ten Thousand Things.

Allow your mind to rest at this point until the urge to inhale prompts your next inhale. Allow inhalation, exhalation, and the two pauses to be of equal duration.

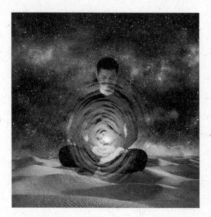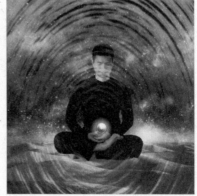

Figure 2.7: Taiji Breathing

The six steps of Taiji breathing are summarized below, followed by the long and short versions of the detailed instruction.

Six-Step Summary:

1. Inhale from the edge of the sphere to Lower Dantian—Yin

2. Breath stops—Wuji

3. Urge to exhale—Dao

4. Exhale to the edge of the sphere—Yang

5. Breath stops—Ten Thousand Things

6. Urge to inhale—Dao

Long version:

1. Adopt Natural Sitting Posture.

2. Envision yourself sitting at the center of a huge sphere. Make this sphere as large as possible without losing your connection to the circumference. The sphere can be a few inches in diameter at first and over time it can expand out millions of miles. This sphere represents the Ten Thousand Things in the Universe. The surface of the sphere represents the leading edge of evolution.

3. Become aware of the entire surface of the sphere and inhale. Draw in the Qi of the Universe toward your Lower Dantian. Draw the energy from above, below, your left side, right side, front side, and back side. Feel the Qi of the Universe converge on Lower Dantian. Concentrate the energy of the Universe at Lower Dantian.

4. In between breaths, become aware of Lower Dantian. This point will eventually transform into the portal that leads to Wuji, your Spirit.

5. Maintain awareness of Lower Dantian until the urge to breathe initiates the exhale. Do not strain. Breathe naturally. Exhale and radiate the concentrated energy from your Lower Dantian toward the circumference of the sphere. Illuminate the Universe with your essence. Feel your energy radiating above, below, to your left side, right side, front side, and back side.

6. Maintain awareness of the sphere until the urge to breathe initiates the exhale. Do not strain. Breathe naturally. Repeat Taiji Breathing nine times or more. Finish the pattern on an inhale and concentrate the energy at Lower Dantian.

7. When you finish practicing, lie down and Nourish your Qi. *I am in Qi; Qi is in me.*

Short Version:

When you become proficient at the long version of Taiji Breathing, you can simplify the exercise by following these instructions:

1. Adopt Natural Sitting Posture.

2. Inhale, draw in Qi to Lower Dantian.

3. Pause.

4. Exhale, radiate Qi to the ends of the Universe.

5. Pause.

6. Repeat nine times or more. Finish the practice on an inhale.

7. Lie down and Nourish your Qi. *I am in Qi; Qi is in me.*

Mystics tend to love reflecting on the wisdom of numbers. The numbers of spirituality are qualitative in nature as opposed to the quantitative numbers used in a spreadsheet or a bill. They represent qualities that arise from the division of wholeness. We showed how these qualitative values can be used to represent the aspects of mind. Though abstract, viewing mind through the filter of number helps us comprehend the integrated wholeness of mind. If you were composing a song, some degree of abstraction would be required to compose the musical score. Musical notes, after all, are mathematical ratios and these ratios hold together the wholeness of the music. But reading sheet music is not the same as hearing the song. To bring the abstraction of music to life requires breathing sound into the notes. Similarly, to elevate the numerical aspects of mind to human proportion, we must give them a voice. That step follows next.

3

Mind as Voice

Taiji in Daily Life

The mental productions of Zero, One, Two, Three, and the Ten Thousand Things play out constantly in our daily lives. At times we are filled with a sense of destiny and at times we fall into nihilistic ruts. At times we are blessed with moments of peace and at times we feel disconnected from the rest of the world. At times we are inspired by benevolence and at times we incline toward malevolence. At times we are guided by higher principles and at times we polarize into conflict. Spirit, Pure Mind, Higher Mind, and Dao each have a distinct voice that break like waves on the shoreline of consciousness.

Maybe you're deliberating an intuition of Spirit, or hanging in the balance of temptation, or miffed and tense about a disagreement. "I won't let her get away with it!" "I'm going to destroy him!" "Should I risk standing up for myself?" "My life feels so empty . . ." The next step in our spiritual journey involves grounding the theory of mind that we developed in the previous chapter into our lived experience. How do you know when Spirit is communicating authentic visions? How do you recognize the temptation of evil? How do you know when your mind is polarized? Learning to recognize the inner voices that govern our internal dialogue and the outer voices that we project out into the world is an essential skill that helps us manage our spiritual journey.

The Voice of Spirit

If we envision Taiji as a compass, the voice of Spirit is the needle that points north. You can spin around and jump up and down, but the needle remains fixed and steady despite the turbulence. The voice that remains steady in moments of adversity, the voice that provides guidance in moments of confusion, the unwavering voice that brings you a sense of peace—these voices are examples of the Voice of Spirit. Imagine that you are lost in the desert and find a satchel that includes a map and a compass. You have been walking in circles and the map indicates that you should head southeast. The compass needle helps you orient and head in a meaningful direction. Before you found the satchel, you were lost. And now you have a clear way forward. When the Voice of Spirit arises in your stream of consciousness, your inner compass needle awakens, and if you follow the path indicated, you develop a clear sense of purpose.

When our choices align with the wisdom of Spirit, we feel a sense of peace. Our actions are unified and coherent. Let's imagine that your name is Ludwig van Beethoven for a moment. You are staring at a blank sheet of music pondering your Fifth Symphony. And then you hear that famous musical phrase, *Ta-Da-Da-Da*. That simple musical phrase is going to guide you throughout the intricate forty-minute composition. Every note you jot down is going to reflect that phrase. If you stray from the essence of those four notes, the composition would lose its integrity. So long as you continue to pull on the thread of those four notes, the music will guide you to perfection.

The Voice of Spirit is like a simple musical phrase. It is efficient and terse yet foundational and absolute. Spirit speaks a few words that may take you months, years, or decades to bring to fruition. The element of time is irrelevant at the level of Spirit because Wuji stands outside of time. Thoughts that emanate from Spirit remain impervious to the passage of time.

When Spirit shapes our inner dialogue, we experience thoughts as absolutely true, and if we ignore their directive, the composition of our life crumbles into incoherent noise. Disconnected from Spirit, we are back in the desert of life wandering around aimlessly and distracting ourselves through the fulfillment of wanton pleasures, fame, and power. When we ignore the voice of Spirit, our words become hollow and heavy. We feel that our life is wasting away. Nihilism—the rejection of meaning and the denial of Spirit—sways the mind toward the predations of evil, polarity, and falsehood. To be clear, religion is incidental to Spirit. An atheist can be spiritual and a priest can be nihilistic. But healthy forms of religion help the mind orient toward Spirit. The sacred religious teachings that transcend time are rooted in the Voice of Spirit, and those teachings inspire the awakening of your Spirit. Some aspects of religion are grounded in culture and opinion, and those parts form the chaff of religious teachings. The timeless truths spoken by spiritual masters who spoke in the Voice of Spirit thousands of years ago remain as relevant today as they will be in a thousand years.

The Voice of Spirit is the voice of creativity. When a mind is aligned with Spirit, creativity overflows. As the mind falls away from Spirit, creativity diminishes. Creativity is not limited to artistic activities. Spirit may inspire you to create a business, to create a daycare center, to create a sports team, to create a nightclub.

Picture yourself wearing a fifty pound suit of armor all day long. Climbing up a staircase feels like a workout. You dread the heaviness of the day, which passes by in slow motion. The Voice of Spirit whispers in your ear and a meaningful vision is revealed. Suddenly, the suit of armor falls away and you feel light. Inertia and gravity fall away. So long as you remain true to your vision, you feel magnetized and are drawn almost effortlessly from one task to another. When your actions align with Spirit you don't tire even when your body is exhausted. You remain absolutely committed to the fulfillment of your creation. Like the proverbial mailman who delivers the mail under all weather conditions, your creative output isn't deterred by adversity, failure, or obstructions. If your excitement abates at the first sign of resistance, that is a sign that you are not aligned with Spirit. You are listening to the directive of a lesser voice.

Imagine that God ushers you into his conference room and sits you down. You are wearing your clunky suit of armor and waddle to the chair uncomfortably.

"My dear friend, I can see that you are feeling miserable at your job," God says.

"It's true, I hate it," you reply.

"If you do this instead, I guarantee you'll be happier." God hands you a memo and your eyes widen as you read it.

"Oh my God, that sounds amazing," you reply.

Let's envision the captain of a tuna fishing vessel standing on the deck of his ship staring out at sea. He has followed the Dao of Tuna Fishing for over three decades and he has mastered the skills of his trade. He knows how the fish think, the waters they like, and the times of day and year they can be caught. He respects the sea and loves his calling. The ship is his home, the open sea is his backyard, and his crew is his family.

Back on shore, a young man is rereading an ad for a position on a tuna vessel. He can't put it down. The newspaper page is folded and he has been carrying it in his back pocket for a week. When he first read it, he didn't think much of it, but he kept on thinking about the opportunity and an inner voice encouraged him to apply for the position. He ignored the voice for some time, but it became louder and louder until he finally relents and calls the number. A gruff voice picks up the line.

"I'm calling about the ad, Captain."

"Alright. Let's meet next Tuesday at the Shark Fin Pub, at three in the afternoon, and we'll talk then."

The young man is sitting at a table at the pub eyeing his watch. It reads 2:58. The captain enters precisely at 3:00 and they shake hands.

"It's a damn hard job," the captain explains. "But it's a damn good job if you're called to do it, and I wouldn't trade it in for the crown of England."

"To be honest, I'm not sure why I'm applying for the job. But I've always felt a strong pull toward the sea, and I can't stop thinking about this opportunity," the young man says.

The captain has a good feeling about this candidate. His gut is telling him that he's the right man for the job and he hires him. The new crew member is committed to learning all that he can about tuna fishing, and he gradually rises up the ranks. Eighteen years pass and he has become an expert at tuna fishing on par with the captain who has become a cherished mentor. When the captain finally decides to retire, he offers to sell the crew member his beloved ship. They shake hands and embrace with tears in their eyes. Within a few weeks, the new captain of the tuna fishing vessel is standing on deck and staring out at sea. He is reflecting on the voice that guided him to the fateful decision that led him to this moment as a profound sense of peace settles over him.

In an alternate universe, the same young man discards the ad and ignores the inner voice. He never calls the captain and instead ends up working as a waiter at the Shark Fin Pub. He befriends the captain and many other sailors that frequent the pub. He listens to their stories about the sea and from time to time, lying in bed, daydreams of being the captain of his own ship.

Spirit graces the mind with a vision. A novel possibility emerges in awareness that feels exciting and frightening at the same time. Spirit is risky. Novelty is risky. Creativity is risky. But if we ignore the voice of Spirit, we are destined to fail. The void intended to be actualized by the vision of Spirit becomes a hole filled with malaise. A sense of foreboding and failure darkens the mood of our life as we literally miss the boat.

Exercise 6: Awaken Your Voice of Spirit

This exercise is intended to help you identify the voice of your Spirit. As you explore this aspect of your mind, consider the following: Can you hear this voice? Do you trust this voice? Will you listen to this voice? The purpose of this exercise is simply to become aware of the messages your Spirit communicates.

1. Assume Natural Sitting Posture.

2. Practice Taiji Breathing for nine cycles.

3. Become aware of the blank screen of awareness in which thoughts arise.

4. Set the intention for your Spirit to reveal itself in the form of a voice or a vision that will fill your life with meaning. Envision a compass needle. Ask your Spirit to point it toward a fulfilling vision. What direction should I follow? What creative energy do you want me to actualize? The revelation of Spirit may be familiar, or it may surprise you.

5. If an authentic vision arises, welcome it and embrace it. If nothing arises, accept the silence graciously. With practice, your connection to Spirit will become stronger over time. Keep on practicing this visualization until you can connect to Spirit and receive guidance almost instantaneously.

6. Nourish your Qi. *I am in Qi; Qi is in me.*

The Voice of Pure Mind

The Voice of Spirit is absolute. The visions emanating from Wuji are not subject to debate or compromise. The message of Spirit is non-negotiable. In Western spiritual traditions, the messages of Spirit are sometimes envisioned as communications delivered by angels. The biblical words for *angel* in ancient Hebrew and Greek literally mean "messenger." The notion is that angels deliver messages originating from the spiritual realm. Angels are not common to Daoist lore, but the notion of an angel can help ground our understanding of spiritual messages in a more familiar framework. A message communicated from the realm of Spirit can be interpreted as an angelic transmission, or as an emanation from Wuji, or even as communication from a deity. Whichever interpretation makes the most sense is the one to embrace as you learn to recognize the interaction between Spirit and Pure Mind in daily life.

Imagine a single man riding the New York City subway minding his own business. He inadvertently makes eye contact with a woman on the train. That instant, he is struck in the heart by Cupid's arrow, an angelic transmission of sorts. He doesn't know this yet, but that woman is destined to become his future spouse, and this chance encounter is going to change his life. They exchange a few words. The few minutes that he shares with her feel otherworldly and larger than life. She gets off at her next station, but she remains present in his thoughts. He has had romantic connections before but this time it feels different. She is not his type, but he can't stop thinking about her. And the more he thinks about her, the more he wants to think about her until her presence becomes a permanent feature in his mind. And at that point, he reaches for his cell phone and texts her. It's fortuitous that he instinctively asked for her number before she got off the train, or else he might be thinking about her for the rest of his life. And it's fortuitous that she uncharacteristically agreed to give him her number. She also felt the call of Spirit to connect with him. The message from Wuji stirred both their heartstrings. An angel gonged their souls. Or maybe the symbolism of Cupid's arrow is more fitting in this instance. Whichever way we choose to dress up the interaction is a matter of personal preference. What isn't a matter of personal preference is the way they feel once the message has been delivered.

Once we are graced with a spiritual message, we are overcome with excitement and some measure of awe. The excitement reflects the deep sense of meaning the vision inspires and the awe reflects the thrill inherent in the change it portends. The messages of Spirit are creative emanations that reshape our lives like invisible hands on a spinning clay pot. They point us in meaningful directions. They invite meaningful experiences and meaningful people into our storylines. The quantity of spiritual messages that an individual receives depends on their openness to Spirit. Wuji is constantly broadcasting messages into our lives, but we may only be receiving a few of those messages with our limited bandwidth. As we strengthen our connection to Spirit, we become attuned to the multitude of spiritual messages that are constantly streaming into our lives.

Some angels are huge and others are tiny. Some messages are monumental, and others are diminutive. All messages add meaning to our day. "Read that book." "Attend this workshop." "Sign up for that yoga class." "Go on that trip." "Speak to this person." "Avoid that person." When we are radically open to Spirit, every moment can be experienced as a spiritual revelation and every moment shines with the promise of spiritual meaning.

Once a spiritual vision is gestating in our mind, it is nourished by the Voice of Pure Mind. The Voice of Pure Mind is the voice of benevolence that feeds the vision of positive energy. The voice of benevolence instills the vision with goodness. Imagine a loving presence whispering in your ear, "You can do it. You can manifest this vision. I love what you are contemplating. It is good and I believe in your success. I sincerely hope that you make it happen." The voice of benevolence is a voice that communicates goodness. It feels good to hear the words spoken by this voice. This voice is benefic. The words are well intentioned. They incline us to embrace the vision fully and to birth the vision by pushing it out into manifestation.

But not all visions end up in a birth. Some spiritual visions are negated by the voice of malevolence. The voice of malevolence is a malicious voice. The voice of malevolence is a destructive voice. Imagine a hateful presence whispering in your ear, "You can't do it. Who are you trying to fool? You're going to hate yourself when you fail. You are not worthy. You don't deserve to succeed. Get that silly idea out of your head before you make a fool of yourself." The voice of malevolence abhors Spirit, goodness, meaning, and peace. Its sole purpose is to destroy goodness and any sense of meaning in your life. It wants to kill your vision and drag you down into a pit of despair.

The voice of benevolence can be communicated from within, or it can be spoken by a benevolent person to whom you open up about your vision. It can be communicated through a spiritual book, a spiritual teacher, or a benefic friend who supports your spiritual growth. Good people will help you actualize your highest good. The benevolent voices are index fingers pointing you toward the high road that leads to spiritual growth and a meaningful life.

The voice of malevolence can be communicated from within, or it can be spoken by a malevolent person to whom you open up about your vision. A malicious voice can come from a jealous friend or a hateful person who doesn't want to see you thrive. If you surround yourself with nefarious people who lack inherent goodness, your social circle will make it difficult for you to create a meaningful life. Malevolent voices are gnarly index fingers pointing us toward the low road that leads to misery and disaster.

The voice of benevolence and the voice of malevolence are mutually exclusive. A choice needs to be made between the two voices as they vie for our attention. Which voice is more powerful? That depends on the quality of your Pure Mind. In the minds of most people, the voices alternate. There is a dialogue between them before a decision is finally made. Free will is the aspect of Pure Mind that considers the arguments between the voices of good and evil like a juror listening to the prosecution and the defense argue their cases.

Let's imagine that Spirit graces a woman with a vision: start your own business by opening a flower shop. The concept fills her with an uplifting sense of meaning. The inner voice of benevolence speaks to her about the goodness of the vision. "A flower shop will fill my life with meaning. I don't like my current job. The people I work with are so competitive and mean. I would love to create beautiful floral arrangements and bring happiness into the lives of others. I deserve to lead a purposeful life and to look forward to Monday mornings. I have some savings, but I am scared of the risk involved. And yet, the vision of my own flower shop is so inspiring, and the more I envision my flower shop, the more the idea grows and the more my heart fills with faith in my eventual success. My father once told me that to find happiness in life, we have to be willing to pay the price of uncertainty. His words are the wind beneath my wings. I meditated and prayed on this vision and my faith in it has grown. I keep hearing an inner voice cheering me on. It tells me that I can succeed if I commit to seeing the vision through. Every day, I get closer and closer to saying yes and acting. I am meeting my sister for dinner tonight and I will open up to her and see what she has to say."

"Get that silly idea out of your mind," the sister says, sipping on a glass of wine. "You have a secure, salaried job with benefits. Are you really going to give it all up just to indulge a childish dream? Grow up, sister. Life is not a fairy tale. Do you really think you 'deserve' to be happy? That myth is for kids. Life is hard and cruel, and you need to be strong enough to bear the misery. Life couldn't care less about your happiness. I'm only saying all of this because I love you and I don't want you to fail. Don't quit your job over a pipe dream. You'll end up broke and unemployed."

As we delve deeper into the mind of the sister, we witness jealousy and malice motivating her words. She is a negative person who would hate to see her sister happy because she is miserable herself. She uses manipulative logic and fear to steer her sister into a life-denying world-view that leads to darkness. She feeds her own sense of power by making her sister feel powerless. Her goal is to destroy the vision, and along with it, the creative spark that would fill her sister's life with meaning. Her goal is to point her sister toward the low road that leads to a gloomy future of hopelessness and despair.

The voice of benevolence and the voice of malevolence are mutually exclusive, and the woman is going to have to make a choice. Does she honor her vision or set it aside? Her free will teeters and totters between the benevolent inner voice that supports the vision and her sister's malevolent words that seek to kill the vision. Which voice is more powerful? Which voice will win? That depends on the quality of the woman's Pure Mind.

The Dao has engineered a reality in which we are free to choose between benevolence and malevolence. We are free to choose good and free to choose evil. We are free to align with Spirit and free to turn our back to Spirit. We are free to bless life and we are free to curse life. Neither benevolence nor malevolence can be imposed. Ultimately, the choice is ours to make as these voices vie for control on the battleground of Pure Mind.

Greater Duality

The realm of Greater Duality is full of light, and it is full of darkness. It is full of benevolence and full of malevolence. The battle between light and darkness is continuously waged inside Pure Mind. Have you ever wished ill of another human being? Have you ever wished failure upon someone that you envy? Have you ever rejoiced at the misfortune of others? Have you ever manipulated or deceived someone just to get ahead?

Has the voice of malevolence ever commandeered your tongue and have you spewed hurtful lies for personal gain? The battle between light and darkness is also continuously waged in the broader world. The face of evil prevails over news feeds. Read the headlines: corrupt leaders stealing resources meant for the underprivileged; dealers peddling deadly drugs to children; gratuitous violence against those who look different; sexual predation and human trafficking; and murderous tyrants oppressing entire populations. Cruelty, terror, and horror await those who follow the low road. Those who incline toward malevolence are empowering evil at their own spiritual peril.

Most of us are caught up in the battle between good and evil. We project benevolence toward some and malevolence toward others. We may be benevolent toward our friends and malevolent toward our enemies and believe that outlook is perfectly normal and healthy. "We are good, and they are evil" is a common refrain. We may project malevolence toward others or even self-destructively toward ourselves. The negative voice that tells us repeatedly that we deserve to be punished, that we deserve to fail, and that we are worthless is self-directed malice. From the perspective of Pure Mind, malevolence directed toward anyone, including ourselves, is never good.

At the ends of the spectrum of Pure Mind are Pure Good and Pure Evil. Pure Good is a mind unable to generate malevolence of any kind toward anyone. Past a certain level of spiritual development, conjuring a negative thought becomes a painful experience. Pure Good only knows benevolence. Sincerely wishing all sentient beings the blessing of peace and the bounty of perfection is the refrain of those souls whose minds have attained Pure Good. At the other extreme of the spectrum lies Pure Evil. A mind abiding in Pure Evil is unable to generate a benevolent thought. Pure Evil knows only malevolence. A sincere disregard for humanity along with an inclination to destroy innocence and the hatred of purity is the driving force behind a mind grounded in Pure Evil.

Without spiritual practice or religious guidance, free will is more likely to incline toward malevolence in the face of adversity. And malevolence can quickly backslide into evil. The judge who hesitates before taking his first bribe will hesitate less the second time around, and will expect a bribe the third time around. *Damned be the innocent!* As a malevolent mind strays deeper into darkness, the voice of conscience fades. Malevolence without conscience gives rise to evil. The guard in the Nazi concentration camp who sleeps soundly at night after leading families into gas chambers is evil. The prison warden who tortures prisoners for fun is evil. When Pure Mind falls prey to extreme malevolence without compunction, it becomes Pure Evil.

As we progress along the spiritual path, we empower our goodness. As we advance spiritually, it becomes harder for our mind to stray into malevolence. At a certain point in our spiritual development, malevolent thoughts become infrequent and painful. As we make our way toward Pure Good, we may stumble from time to time, and in those instances, our conscience will remind us of our lapse through the feeling of guilt. The sting of guilt alerts Pure Mind that it has crossed the line into malevolence. And this reminder is like a rubber band that snaps the mind back toward benevolence and goodness.

Experientially, benevolence is measured by our capacity to bless, and malevolence is measured by our capacity to curse. Imagine that the person whom you love the most is going away on a perilous journey. At the moment of parting, you bless their journey. The feeling of a blessing is different than the feeling of love or any other emotion. You can love someone and bless them, but you can also bless a stranger with whom you have no personal connection. The key to blessing anyone is an open heart, but an open heart is not enough. While love is connected to the heart, a blessing emanates from the top of the head, the crown. When we bless someone, we feel a sacred energy emanating through us from above. Our capacity for benevolence is rooted in the connection that we cultivate between our heart and the top of our head.

Malevolence is rooted in a wounded heart. When someone hurts us directly or indirectly, our heart shuts down. Have you ever hated someone that you once loved? When love turns to hate, benevolence transforms into malevolence. When our heart shatters and turns to stone, it's unable to connect with the top of our head and we are unable to generate benevolent thoughts. Any violation or betrayal that hardens the heart can drive the mind to extreme malevolence. The subversion of the natural order through horrors such as murder, rape, corruption, racism, and betrayal can breed a deep hatred. Our wounds can lash out at one person, a group of people, or even the entire world. Like love, hatred knows no bounds. But malevolence can also transform into benevolence when there is healing, forgiveness, and redemption. Once the heart heals, it can reconnect with the sacredness at the top of the head and recapture the capacity to bless.

Malevolence can revert to benevolence through an act of redemption. Redemption arises when conscience resurges in a malevolent mind and draws that mind back toward goodness. The former gang member who devotes his life to saving street kids from a life of criminality is an example of redemption. Any kind of meaningful sacrifice can transform malevolence into benevolence. If a malevolent mind does not choose the path of redemption but continues along the low road, that mind can become subservient to negative otherworldly beings that are described in the teachings of Buddhism, Hinduism, Christianity, Judaism, and Islam, as well as Daoism. Authentic spiritual teachers and religions warn against the power of evil and only the ignorant turn a blind eye to those warnings.

Daoist sages took the danger of evil very seriously. An entire branch of Daoist religion is devoted to protecting against evil. Daoists recognized the destructive powers of negativity that spread mayhem and chaos. They also recognized that the low road is a dead end, because ultimately the path to Spirit is closed to malevolent minds. Evil can never know peace or perfection. It is doomed to destroy everything and anything, including itself.

Daoist sages created mediation practices to empower Pure Mind and offer individuals a clear path toward Spirit. As we progress spiritually, malevolence becomes increasingly disgusting. Would you eat excrement from a plate made of gold? As we empower benevolence, we are repelled by malevolence despite the seductive lures it uses to manipulate the mind.

In all the years I was with my master, Xiao Yao, I never witnessed even the slightest hint of malevolence. He embodied pure goodness. To be in the presence of such an individual is spiritually transformative. Once you understand that a human being can be supremely benevolent, that individual becomes an endless source of inspiration that accelerates your own spiritual advancement. Finding a living spiritual teacher or even one that is no longer incarnate but who has left behind a legacy of spiritual wisdom is an invaluable blessing on your journey to Spirit.

Exercise 7: Awaken Free Will

Where on this spectrum of Pure Mind is your mind centered? Do you spend more time contemplating benefic thoughts or malefic thoughts? The following exercise, Awaken Free Will, is intended to help you recognize the voice of benevolence and the voice of malevolence as they arise in your mind. Wherever you fall on the spectrum between good and evil, know that the practices prescribed in this book will guide your Pure Mind toward benevolence and goodness and eventually toward the perfection of Spirit.

1. Assume Natural Sitting Posture.

2. Practice Taiji Breathing for a series of nine cycles.

3. Become aware of the blank screen of awareness in which thoughts arise. Awaken awareness.

4. Become aware of someone in your life who has been good to you. Become aware of any benevolent thoughts that arise as you consider this person.

5. Become aware of someone in your life who has caused you intentional harm. Become aware of any malevolent thoughts that arise in your mind as you consider this person.

6. Invoke your free will, the aspect of your mind that can witness impartially. Is your inclination toward benevolence greater than your inclination toward malevolence? Are you more likely to bless or to curse? Take an honest assessment of your Pure Mind. The purpose of this exercise is to recognize

and distinguish between the two voices and realize their relative strength.

7. Become aware of the person who has been good to you again. Become aware of the benevolent thoughts that arise as you consider this person. Bless this person.

8. Nourish your Qi. *I am in Qi; Qi is in me.*

The Voice of Higher Mind

A pivotal election is going to take place tomorrow. Two political parties are vying for dominance and power. Half the nation leans toward one political party and the other half leans toward the other party. One side believes in freedom and the other side believes in equality. One believes in the rights of the individual and the other believes in communal rights. One believes in self-sufficiency and the other believes in social welfare. One believes in severity against criminals and the other believes in leniency. Each side is wagging fingers at the other side, "We are right, and you are wrong. No, you are wrong, and we are right."

While issues centering on good and evil have bipartisan support, issues centering on right and wrong become polarized. If a judge is corrupt, for example, both sides of the political divide would agree that that judge should be castigated regardless of their political inclination. But if you consider electing a liberal or conservative judge, two sides will polarize over the issue. Daoist sages made a distinction between Greater Duality and Lesser Duality. Greater Duality represents the unflinching divide between good and evil. Lesser Duality, on the other hand, represents the line constantly wavering between right and wrong. Not too long ago it was wrong for women to vote. Now it is right. Nowadays it would be wrong to question many issues that were right a generation or two ago. The line between right and wrong differs across cultures and epochs. This line is relative and subject to continual change. In fact, it must change in order to enable societies to adapt to new realities.

Two men are seated together on a five-hour flight. One man upholds views that are diametrically opposed to the other man's views. One is staunchly conservative and the other is staunchly liberal. They strike up a conversation that quickly veers into politics, and before long, a political debate is taking place at thirty thousand feet. To their surprise, each man is raising interesting points. At each turn of the conversation, their opposing perspectives are being stretched and the dialogue is deepening their understanding. By the time the plane lands, they have discovered common ground on which compromise is possible. They exit the plane and shake hands with mutual respect.

That is one scenario that could play out. But there is another possible outcome, this one messy and disruptive. In this scenario, the discussion gets heated, fiery language is exchanged as the two men raise their voices over each other to the consternation of the other passengers. Polarization can lead to conflict and even violence. Those outcomes can unfold on an airplane or anywhere else human beings congregate. Entire nations can polarize, segments within a population can polarize, communities can polarize, families can polarize, two individuals can polarize, and we can even polarize within ourselves. Humans have polarized throughout history, and we remain polarized today. Technological advances do not appear to mitigate polarization, and arguably, they exacerbate polarization as faster communication speeds up conflict between larger swaths of people in real time.

Polarization is a central feature of social interaction. Place any group of individuals in any setting and before long they will divide. At first, we might think that polarity is unhealthy since it can lead to argumentation and conflict, but consider the alternative—autocracy. Whenever dissent and opposition are disallowed in a social setting, tyranny ensues. Giving an individual or group absolute power without any checks and balances opens the door to evil. If an evil leader wanted to create an evil empire, the first thing that individual would do is demonize dissent. Autocratic leaders repress opposition. A social order that disallows dissent is eventually going to follow the low road that leads to terror and horror. Think of the Pure Evil perpetrated by the Nazis in Germany, the Stalinists in Russia, and the Khmer Rouge in

Cambodia, where even the slightest opposition was met by concentration camps, gulags, or bullets.

Polarity is not evil. Polarity protects against evil. Polarity is a natural and healthy social dynamic that prevents autocrats and tyrannies from gaining control. Both sides of an argument bring awareness to social issues that need to be addressed. Both sides are inextricably linked like the front and the back of a coin. Polarity draws awareness. If you wanted to raise awareness about a particular issue, you would need to create opposition. Oppositions are the fertile ground where change can happen.

If you want to play tennis, you need more than a racket and a ball. You need another player on the opposite side of the court. You serve the ball and they hit it back over the net. That back and forth continues until someone wins the volley. Sometimes you lose the point and sometimes you win the point, but you both improve your game by competing against each other. The polarity that arises on the tennis court arises more broadly in any social context. Through polarity in politics, society improves its game. Through polarity in a relationship, the partnership improves its game. Opposition makes us better tennis players in any social context.

When polarities are integrated, balance and harmony ensue and everyone benefits. But polarities can also express themselves in unhealthy ways. The tension between two sides can devolve into violence. Unhealthy polarity destabilizes growth and disrupts development. When the two tennis players are hitting each other over the head with their tennis rackets, they are likely to injure each other so that they can no longer play and improve their game.

Antagonism between opposing sides is responsible for many bloody conflicts around the world. Think of a soccer world championship where fans of both sides hurl insults at each other. Now imagine handing those fans swords. It wouldn't take very long for those two sides to wage a medieval-style battle on the playing field. How many of the wars that we read about in history books were started by hot-headed, polarized conflicts? Good people on opposite ends of a polarity can become antagonistic and precipitate terrible conflict. Benevolent people can lose their minds when they are antagonized. Goodness is not enough to prevent violence.

Unhealthy polarization can lead to physical violence, and it can lead to emotional violence. We can punch another person in the nose with our fist or bruise their dignity with our mouth. We can lob nasty insults at each other. We can have yelling matches and speak hurtful words. And this kind of violence can be perpetrated by two otherwise benevolent individuals. Most worrisome is the danger that polarized violence can incline a benevolent mind toward evil. Violence can easily incite malevolence. Disagreement can deteriorate into hatred.

Evil adores violence. It relishes the idea of sneaking into a benevolent mind in a moment of extreme polarization and pushing goodness over the edge. In a moment of polarized rage, a good husband might raise his hand and strike his wife. Or a good mother might hit her child. And if antagonism can incline a benevolent mind toward violence, consider what antagonism does to a malevolent mind. Imagine two malevolent and antagonistic gangs in a deadly confrontation. Horrific acts of shameless cruelty would ensue.

Daoist sages investigating the nature of duality recognized the danger of unhealthy polarity. They looked for a method to prevent polarity from becoming antagonistic and backsliding into evil. Daoist sages reasoned that the polarized mind is unsettled and tense. It is restless and uneasy. It is exhausted and drained by argumentation and dissent. Their brilliant insight was that every polarity secretly seeks integration. The integration of polarities resolves contention, advances the agendas of both sides, and leads to balance and harmony.

Picture a five-pound stick that you must carry around all day long. You try holding it by one end and after a few minutes you get tired. Then you switch to the other end, but that doesn't help. You change your grip and grasp it along the middle. Two and a half pounds on one side balances two and a half pounds on the other side. It's much easier to carry a heavy weight when it is properly balanced. Now, place that stick on the ground and place a fulcrum at the midpoint where you were holding it.

You have created a scale. You can use this stick to weigh one thing against another and find the point of balance.

Higher Mind is the aspect of mind that acts like that fulcrum. It seeks the balance point between polarities. It integrates polarities and diffuses tension and violence. When we abide in Higher Mind, we no longer identify with one side or the other. We no longer grab the stick by one end or the other. When we abide in Higher Mind, we identify with the fulcrum point that balances opposition and harmonizes discord.

Imagine a heated debate between two candidates running for office. One says up and the other says down. One says left and the other says right. One says always and the other says never. The tension between the two is palpable and the audience is on edge. Everyone feels the imbalance and discord. Who is right and who is wrong? We pause the fiery exchange and invite a Daoist sage onto the debate stage.

"Madam, what do you think?" the moderator asks. The sage, operating from Higher Mind replies, "Both candidates are partially right and partially wrong. Rather than attacking each other they could work together to create better policies. Integrating the two extremes leads to superior resolutions that foster balance and harmony. Each candidate must be willing to step into the shoes of the other and embrace what is right about the opposing perspective and reject what is wrong about their own. When you see things through the eyes of the other, and the other sees things through your eyes, balance and harmony can be established. But the integration of opposites can only happen when both sides show goodwill. Without goodwill, a polarity can never be resolved."

What is goodwill? Goodwill is the quality created by Higher Mind. Goodwill is made up of higher principles, or moral principles, that facilitate integration. Imagine that you are arguing with another person. Do you respect the opposing point of view? Are you considerate? Are you fair-minded? Are you willing to concede parts of an argument if you are proven wrong? Are you willing to discuss differences without imposing your will? Are you more interested in creating balance and harmony than in being right and proving the other side wrong?

If you are arguing with someone who is showing you goodwill, you feel seen and understood. You sense higher principles driving the conversation forward. You sense moral principles holding the dialogue together. When two opposing sides both express goodwill, polarities are usually resolved efficiently. Disagreements lead to better policies. Arguments lead to more efficient solutions. Dissent leads to fairer outcomes. With mutual goodwill, the integration of opposites arises naturally, and balance and harmony are established without requiring much effort. With goodwill, polarity averts antagonism and violence.

Imagine two parents arguing over their style of childrearing. The father is advocating for severity to teach their son self-sufficiency, resilience, and strength, while the mother is advocating for leniency to teach their son mercy, forgiveness, and tolerance. Who is right and who is wrong? The father argues that the world is harsh and, at times, unforgiving, and that their son needs to learn how to survive in that environment. The father is right. Sometimes, the world favors those with thick skin. The mother argues that without mercy, a person can become cruel and heartless. Mercy and forgiveness open the heart and allow for love to be given and received. The mother is also right. The inability to experience mercy can make someone cold-blooded. Should the son grow up to be thick-skinned and heartless or thin-skinned and loving?

Without goodwill, this argument might last indefinitely with each side digging in deeper. With goodwill, the father and mother can acknowledge each other's concern and agree to a style of childrearing that integrates toughness and kindness. With goodwill, they can realize that they both care for the boy in different ways. The mutual care underlying the polarity of parenting becomes the fulcrum of integration. The parents can encourage the boy to face challenges and strive for success on his own merit, and show the boy kindness rather than punishment when he fails to achieve his goal. Whatever happens, care remains constant. With parental care, the boy can develop thick skin and an open heart. In this example, care is the fulcrum that integrates the polarity between toughness and love. Care is the higher principle that integrates the opposition between severity and leniency.

Higher Mind is the aspect of your mind that can identify the higher principle needed to resolve a polarity. There are a limited number of higher principles and each one of them is an effective fulcrum in a specific context. The national motto of France is *Liberty, Equality, and Fraternity.* Liberty and equality are opposites, and fraternity represents the fulcrum of integration between this polarity. Fraternity, or more broadly humanity, is the higher principle that keeps balance and harmony between the polarities. Liberty, Equality, and Care does not feel like the right formulation. And fraternity does not feel like the appropriate fulcrum for childrearing either. Higher Mind can hone in on the right higher principle needed to integrate a given polarity.

The list of higher principles includes courage, reliability, consistency, productivity, clarity, care, safety, nobility, discernment, efficiency, fairness, kindness, honesty, righteousness, caution, integrity, authenticity, humanity, and compassion. Each of these higher principles transcends polarity. Each side of a polarity can embrace any of these higher principles without forgoing their views. And with goodwill and the right higher principle, polarity can be integrated, and tension can resolve into balance and harmony.

But what happens when one of the opposing parties is malevolent and mired in ill will? Ill will is the rejection of high-minded principles in the pursuit of raw power. Ill will doesn't care about right or wrong. Ill will cares only about domination and supremacy. Ill will wants to silence the opposition and kill dissent. Ill will is the spawn of malevolence and strives to drive polarity into chaos, mayhem, and destruction.

When goodwill and ill will oppose each other, the same principle we previously discussed applies. The side that embraces benevolence and goodwill must invoke a higher principle that will dispel ill will. Ill will and malevolence thrive on deception, manipulation, temptation, seduction, and lies. If goodwill perseveres through the storm of negativity, the discord and disharmony of ill will and malevolence will be exposed, and negativity will retreat. Consider a beautiful piece of music and nails scratching a blackboard. Which would you rather listen to? When ill will is exposed, the discord it embodies drives people away. When ill will is exposed, it destroys itself from within.

Daoist sages understood that ultimately benevolence overpowers malevolence, and that, paradoxically, malevolence and ill will ultimately strengthen benevolence and goodwill. Positivity is strengthened by the negativity it overcomes. The sages developed spiritual practices intended to strengthen benevolence and goodwill because light obliterates darkness. These practices will be shared in the coming chapters.

Exercise 8: Awaken Goodwill

This exercise is meant to draw awareness to your capacity for goodwill. By exercising goodwill, you invoke Higher Mind and the moral principles that lead to balance and harmony.

1. Assume Natural Sitting Posture.

2. Practice Taiji Breathing for a series of nine cycles.

3. Become aware of the blank screen of awareness in which thoughts arise.

4. Become aware of an argument you are having or have had recently with another person.

5. Imagine that this person is arguing their point in a foreign language that you do not understand. Since you do not comprehend the words, you are not offended by them.

6. Listen to the voice of this person with respect. Let them feel your consideration as they express their point of view. Let them finish what they have to say without interrupting them.

7. Now imagine that it is your turn to express your opinion in a language that they do understand. Express your ideas without imposing your will. Speak in a measured way. Be clear in the arguments that you present. Focus on why you think that you are right, not on why you think that the other side is wrong.

8. Now, step into the shoes of the other person and repeat the exercise. Articulate their perspective as clearly as you can.

9. When you are able to experience the same level of respect and consideration expressing both sides of the argument, you have awakened your goodwill.

10. Set an intention. The next time I get into a polarized situation, I will awaken goodwill and observe how the discussion unfolds with the utmost respect and consideration.

11. Nourish your Qi. *I am in Qi; Qi is in me.*

The Voice of Practical Mind

A benevolent man full of goodwill pulls up at a mechanic shop. His engine is making a troubling sound. The mechanic lifts the hood to examine the engine. His arms are tattooed with serpents that run up his neck and cover his cheeks with menacing fangs. The mechanic emanates an ominous presence. Inwardly, this man is malevolent and brimming with ill will.

"Run the engine, I want to hear the sound," he says.

The benevolent man turns the engine on, and it lets out a coughing sound.

"There's about ten bad sounds a car like yours makes when she's unhappy, and your troubled child has a clogged fuel filter," the mechanic says.

"It's remarkable that you can diagnose the problem just by listening to the engine noise."

"They don't call me the car whisperer for no reason," the mechanic replies.

Malevolence and ill will do not preclude technical competence and skill. A benevolent person may be competent or incompetent and a malevolent person can be competent or incompetent. Anyone can become a car whisperer, or a computer repair whisperer, or a guitar whisperer, or a carpentry whisperer if they put the time into developing a skill set. Competence and skill in any field fall under the influence of

Practical Mind. You can be a great car mechanic despite your negativity. In the realm of leaky roofs, tax returns, website design, and all the other needs that require servicing, what matters most is your skill level. When dealing with practical matters, we want competent people servicing our needs and solving our problems. We don't need to interview the electrician repairing our electrical panel. All we need to know is that they are qualified to do the work. If you were placing your child in daycare, the high-mindedness and benevolence of the teachers would matter. But if you're hiring a contractor to pave your driveway, does it make a difference either way? We get quotes from several qualified contractors and usually settle on the lowest price.

Practical Mind seeks competence and skillfulness in others and practical mind helps us develop our own competence and skillfulness. We tend to become good at what we like. If we like to solve certain kinds of problems, we are likely to develop skills and become competent in that field. Practical Mind divides the world into likes and dislikes. It pursues likes and avoids dislikes. Practical Mind improves at a skill by following what is true and avoiding what is false, and by doing what is correct and avoiding what is incorrect. There is a correct way to repair a clogged drainpipe and an incorrect way. The correct way includes any method that solves the problem efficiently. The incorrect way does not solve the problem. At the level of Practical Mind, solving problems is what matters most.

What mattered most to the Practical Minds of Daoist sages was to develop a methodology to solve the problem of human suffering. Cars can break down and so can the human bodymind. Cars can make troubling sounds and so do human beings. We complain about this problem or that problem. *I have a headache. My lower back hurts. I am an angry person. I am addicted to gambling. I hate myself.* The troubled sounds that we make when we are unhappy were the practical concern of Daoist sages. They became experts at repairing the human bodymind. They were "human whisperers." They used herbs, acupuncture, and lifestyle changes to help address chronic disease. They developed Qigong movement exercises to help prevent degenerative diseases. And they developed meditation practices to address the problem of human suffering.

As human beings, we experience loss, betrayal, disease, and death on an order of magnitude not experienced by other lifeforms. When we are broken by life, and to some degree we are all broken, how do we heal? The repair of the human condition was the problem Daoist sages set about to solve. And their solution to this problem was to develop a series of meditation practices that define the spiritual journey.

The spiritual journey begins wherever we are. Our spirit may be broken. We may waver in and out of benevolence. Our morals may be open to question. Daoist meditation practices can guide us from the present moment, wherever we are situated existentially, all the way to perfection and beyond. My spiritual master took me in as a disciple when I was eight years old and led me to the heights of spiritual achievement within a few years of serious practice. Becoming competent at spirituality usually takes a few years of serious practice, just like any other skill set. For some it takes longer, for others it takes shorter. Once you set a clear intention and initiate the process, trust the process. You can't force grass to grow by pulling on it. Allow your spiritual nature to unfold organically, however long it takes.

Learning to relax your body by shaking off excess tension is helpful when you are preparing your body for meditation practice. I encourage you to embrace movement exercises to release any excess tension that you are holding. Our bodies and our minds are intermeshed. When we experience mental tension, we tense our bodies unconsciously. The mental tension can dissipate, but if our bodies continue to hold the tension, we remain on edge. Releasing physical tension is a powerful way to also release mental tension, and since meditation is a process that spans the mental realm from Practical Mind to Spirit and Dao, having a pliable and relaxed bodymind is important. When your bodymind is in a relaxed state, you will be drawn to meditation and the journey will proceed smoothly. Your bodymind needs to be relaxed and you also need to feel comfortable sitting down for extended periods of time. Skeletal alignment and the ability to maintain postural integrity are as important as having a relaxed bodymind. It doesn't matter what practice you choose to relax your bodymind and align your skeletal structure. What matters is that sitting doesn't become an obstacle to meditating.

Once your mind is free of tension and your body is comfortable in Natural Sitting Posture, your vehicle is ready for the journey. The practices taught in this book are intended to guide you from Higher Mind all the way to Spirit. There are three main practices that are taught. The Six Healing Sounds, presented in chapter 5, is a practice intended to develop Higher Mind and awaken higher principles. Through this practice, you strengthen your goodwill and moral character.

The second practice, Twelve Meridian Empowerment, is presented in chapter 6. The Meridian Empowerment is intended to develop Pure Mind and awaken your benevolence. Through this practice, you strengthen your power to bless and purify your mind.

The third practice, Huo Lu Gong Spirit Cultivation, is presented in chapter 7. Huo Lu Gong is a practice intended to develop Spirit and awaken Perfect Peace. Through this practice, you extinguish desire and abide in a sublime state of serenity. There are more advanced practices that Daoist sages developed to cultivate Spirit and awaken Dao and those will be shared at some future point.

Exercise 9: Three Dantian Taiji Breathing

In further preparation for your journey, I would like to introduce one more exercise that builds on two exercises we have already practiced, Exercise 2—Chanting Ong, Ah, Hong—and Exercise 5—Taiji Breathing. Three Dantian Taiji Breathing incorporates these two other practices. The purpose of this exercise is to concentrate more Qi energy at the Three Dantians in anticipation of the practices presented in the next three chapters.

1. Assume Natural Sitting Posture.

2. Practice Taiji Breathing at the Upper Dantian for nine or more cycles.

3. Chant Ong, *ongggg* . . . to energize the Upper Dantian three or more times.

4. Practice Taiji Breathing at the Middle Dantian for nine or more cycles.

5. Chant Ah, ahhhhh . . . to energize the Middle Dantian three or more times.

6. Practice Taiji Breathing at the Lower Dantian for nine or more cycles.

7. Chant Hong, honggg . . . to energize the Lower Dantian three or more times.

8. Chant Ong, Ah, Hong three or more times to activate the Three Dantians and the Central Meridian. Feel the sound vibration travel along the central axis of your body.

9. Nourish your Qi. *I am in Qi; Qi is in me.*

The Voice of Dao

One, Two, Three, Ten Thousand. Spirit, Pure Mind, Higher Mind, Practical Mind. Peace, benevolence, goodwill, competence and nihilism, malevolence, ill will, and incompetence. From where do all of these realms and qualities arise? What holds the space for all experience to manifest? In this reality of ours, at this very moment, sublime goodness and atrocious horror are being enacted somewhere. Birth and death are happening simultaneously. The entirety of human experience is unfolding in real time. What is the wholeness that is creating the space for all experience to arise? What is the wholeness that holds the riverbed of time? What is the wholeness that is creating space for not just human experience but animal, plant, and mineral experience. What is the wholeness that is creating space for the experience of a school of fish caught in a tidal wave and the frozen glaciers on Jupiter's moon Europa. What is the wholeness that is holding space for the experience of a first kiss and a final farewell.

The wholeness that creates space for all experience transcends *experience*. The wholeness that creates space for all existence transcends *existence*. The wholeness that creates space for all things is nothing. The wholeness that includes beginnings and endings has no beginning and no end. The wholeness that creates the space for Creation is uncreated. The wholeness that creates time is timeless. The wholeness that creates the space for all knowledge is unknowable. The wholeness that holds the space for the fullness of all is empty. The wholeness that holds the space for all being is nonbeing. That wholeness is called Dao.

Your experience is a part of a grand event. You stand at the center of everything. Every thought, feeling, and action that arises from your being arises in the emptiness of Dao. Your benevolence and malevolence arise in the emptiness of Dao. Your Spirit and perfection arise in the emptiness of Dao. Your goodwill and ill will arise in the emptiness of Dao. Your competence and incompetence arise in the emptiness of Dao. Your existence arises in the emptiness of Dao.

Dao is nameless because it is neither subject nor object. It cannot be reduced to a noun, verb, adverb, adjective, or preposition. Dao transcends the elements of language. Grammar cannot grasp Dao. Dao cannot be grasped by the hands or the mind, and yet it grasps all things. It is grasping your mind right now. It is grasping this moment. The emptiness grasping your being is Dao.

Dao opens the space for growth, development, and evolution. Dao enables time and space to open up to change. The sense of destiny that drives Spirit into manifestation is Dao. The sense of possibilities that opens a path to novelty is Dao. The vacuum that Spirit fills with creativity is Dao. The void that enables free will to emerge is Dao. The fulcrum that allows for the integration of opposites is Dao. The space in which competence can arise is Dao. Dao is the membrane of emptiness that surrounds every facet of experience at every level of existence. Dao is The Way of All Ways.

Daoist sages mapped out a spiritual path that enables Spirit to reunite with Dao. This process is a high altitude path that is open to all but that few travel. The reunion of perfection with wholeness transforms Spirit. When Spirit awakens as Dao, Spirit abides in wholeness. When Spirit awakens as Dao, Spirit can walk the earth. When Spirit awakens as Dao, wholeness can enter space-time and perfection can shake your hand. The mind that awakens as Dao embodies stillness in action. The spiritual master who abides as Dao has transcended the laws of time and space. This individual has the ability to perform miracles, change destiny, and transform the laws of karma. The spiritual master transcends life and death, sleep and wakefulness, consciousness and unconsciousness. The mind that abides as Dao is immortal, extinguished, transfigured, and merged with God. Some call this individual an Immortal, a Boddhisatva, or a Saint. The names and titles are meaningless to these individuals. What is meaningful to them and fuels their sense of destiny is that you discover the Dao that leads to the Dao. The Great Dao, the Dao of all Daos, is our shared destiny as humans.

Dao is ever-present, and in a human being, Dao manifests as awareness itself. Your awareness is emptiness. Awareness lacks qualities and opens up space for all qualities. Awareness is formless and opens up space for all forms. Awareness is like water that takes on all forms and flavors, though it lacks form and flavor. Your awareness opens up the space that is contained by your experience. Your best and your worse moments arise in formless awareness. Your sense of destiny arises in formless awareness. Your spiritual urges arise in formless awareness. Your free will arises in formless awareness. Your higher principles arise in formless awareness. Your competence arises in formless awareness. Your being arises in formless awareness. The Universe arises in empty formless awareness. Awareness is Dao. Bringing awareness to your spiritual practice is the way to invite Dao into your spiritual journey. In every exercise in this book, you will notice the words, "become aware . . ." These words are an invocation of Dao.

The Voice of Dao is the emptiness that creates the space for all other voices to be expressed. The space that opens up around radiant benevolence and warm-hearted goodwill is the Voice of Dao. The space that opens up around spine curling malevolence and hot-headed ill will is also the Voice of Dao. The space that opens up around your next thought or emotion is the Voice of Dao. The space that opens up around your next breath is the Voice of Dao. The Voice of Dao is the silent emptiness that allows all voices to emerge. The Voice of Dao is the great stage on which the performance of life unfolds.

Emptiness is neither one nor many, and yet it is also both. Emptiness is neither this nor that, but it is also both. Emptiness is neither now nor later, but it is also both. Emptiness is everything and nothing. And the wholeness of emptiness connects everything to everything else. If you love someone and they love you back, the love that you share is connected through the emptiness of Dao. If you fear someone and they are angry at you, the fear and the anger are connected through the emptiness of Dao. The wholeness of Dao connects one thing to everything and everything to one thing. It connects all things to nothing and nothing to all things. The activity of your mind that arises in emptiness is experienced by the emptiness of Creation, so that at the level of Dao, your thoughts, feelings, and actions are in constant contact with the thoughts, feelings, and actions of all other human beings.

The invisible network of emptiness opens up space for synchronicities to arise as these mental forms interact. Synchronicities are meaningful coincidences that appear to have no causal relationship. You think of an old friend, and she calls you the next day. You are looking for a rare book and you find it in some random bookstore. You want to travel to Machu Picchu, and you meet someone at some random dinner party who lives there. Synchronicities are expressions of Dao. As awareness of Dao awakens, these sorts of connections become more prevalent and at a certain point in our spiritual development, synchronicities stream into our lives with regularity.

As Dao opens in your life, a sense of effortless flow characterizes the way in which events unfold. When you awaken the emptiness of a thought, thinking becomes non-thinking. When you awaken the emptiness of an action, action becomes non-action. When you awaken the emptiness of your being, being becomes nonbeing. The non-thinking and non-action of your nonbeing leads to the effortless accomplishment of all things. When you awaken as emptiness, effort becomes effortless. Daoist sages called this Wu Wei, non-doing. Wu Wei is trusting Dao to lead the way.

With each step of the spiritual journey, we invoke Dao and open up space for Wu Wei to guide our destiny. With each mindful breath we take, we open up space for Wu Wei to lead with effortless flow. With each action that we take with awareness, we open up space for Wu Wei to provoke synchronicities and create new connections.

Dao is the permanent solution to the existential crisis of being human. The crisis of suffering, disease and death, the crisis of loss and betrayal, the crisis of disasters and catastrophes, the crisis of divine injustice, and all the other incomprehensible traumas that bruise the soul. Those crises are resolved with permanent finality when a human being becomes a child of Dao.

With each stage of spiritual accomplishment, distinct virtues arise. At the level of Practical Mind, the virtues of competence arise. At the level of Higher Mind, the virtues of goodwill arise. At the level of Pure Mind, the virtues of benevolence arise. At the level of Spirit, the virtues of perfection arise. At the level of Dao, the virtues of Wu Wei arise. As we progress spiritually, our minds are endowed with these virtues in greater frequency and magnitude. The space between moments of doubt grows narrower and thinner until we finally return home to Dao, and all discontent is extinguished.

As we travel the Way of Virtue, we open to the sublime and terrifying experience of being human. Being human is the toughest job in Creation and the most precious gift. At least on this planet, no other species possesses the mental capacity to reunite with the Supreme Ultimate. Consider yourself blessed to lead this difficult life. Given the countless lifeforms that populate this world, we represent the tiny handful that can travel the Way of Virtue and abide in the perfection of wholeness. Make that blessing count!

Exercise 10: Awaken Awareness

In this exercise, we are going to become aware of awareness itself. As awareness expands, we connect more fully to Dao. As awareness grows, the Voice of Dao becomes more palpable, and we are able to fill emptiness with the fullness of all our other voices.

1. Assume Natural Sitting Posture.

2. Open your eyes and become aware of some aspect of your external environment. Perhaps an object or a sound, or the feeling of the floor or the chair on which you sit. Perhaps the temperature in the room. The feeling of your clothes on your skin.

3. Close your eyes and become aware of some aspect of your internal environment. Perhaps a feeling or a memory that comes to mind.

4. Keep your eyes closed and become aware of some aspect of your external environment once again.

5. Open your eyes and become aware of some aspect of your internal environment once again.

6. Keep your eyes open and become aware of awareness, the space in which the objective world and the subjective world both arise.

7. Close your eyes and become aware of awareness, the space in which the objective world and the subjective world both arise.

8. Awaken awareness and become aware of the emptiness of your mind that enables all the voices in your head to manifest.

9. Nourish your Qi. *I am in Qi; Qi is in me.*

In the pages leading up to this one, we explored the aspects of mind through the abstraction of number: Zero, One, Two Three, and Ten Thousand. We gave each of those numbers a voice and explored the kinds of qualities produced by the aspects of mind. In the pages that follow, we link the aspects of mind to aspects of the body. Have you ever gotten drunk? Then you know that the body and the mind are insepa-rable bedfellows. Where the body goes, the mind follows. Conversely, where the mind goes, the body follows. We can leverage our minds to transform our body. This latter principle highlights the reasoning under-lying Qigong meditation practice. As you shall soon see, the body can also get drunk on Spirit.

4

Mind as Body

We are Bodyminds

One of the defining features of the Daoist worldview is the notion that we are bodyminds, which is to say that the aspects of the mind that we have been exploring correlate to aspects of our body. Practical Mind, for example, is correlated with the skeletal muscles and their related soft tissue that control the voluntary movement of our limbs and breath. Qigong movement exercises are an expression of Practical Mind, as they rely on the repeated movement of our limbs in coordination with our breath. Through Qigong movement practice, we enhance the well-being of the body and develop improved circulation, joint lubrication, Qi flow, skeletal alignment, and body awareness.

There are many types of Qigong movement exercises. Some strive to calm the nervous system and balance energies through slow movement. Some strengthen soft tissue. Some coordinate body unity to generate power. Some Qigong movement practices are soft and yielding while others are hard. One practice known as Iron Palm transforms the soft tissue and bones of the hands and forearms, making them robust weapons able to break through stones with impunity. With enough discipline and effort, anyone can develop impressive Qigong skills. Practicing Qigong movement exercises, however, does not impart moral character or develop higher principles. Many bandits and thugs mastered Qigong skills and attained a high level of proficiency in the martial arts. Hitting a bag filled with iron pellets repeatedly makes your punching power fearsome, but it doesn't cultivate moral character.

Qigong movement exercises prepare the physical body for the practice of Qigong meditations that cultivate the other aspects of mind. In this sense, they are necessary but not sufficient to help us travel the spiritual path that leads to Spirit. Each aspect of mind that we explored previously is cultivated by a specific meditation that focuses on different parts of the energy body. As we awaken those parts of our energy body, we awaken the corresponding aspect of the mind.

The spiritual path that we will follow in *The Way of Virtue* tracks a progression that leads from Higher Mind to Pure Mind to Spirit. Each aspect of mind is cultivated through a specific meditation practice, and each practice serves as the foundation for the next. Higher Mind is cultivated through a meditation practice associated with the Internal Organs. The network of Organs defines the domain of Higher Mind. I can ask you to wiggle your small finger, but are you able to wiggle your gallbladder? Skeletal muscles are subject to voluntary control, but those muscles are unable to access deep structures like the Internal Organs. Activating the Internal Organs that are situated inside the core of the body requires a meditative approach that does not rely on physical movement. The meditation practice that activates the Organs uses sound resonance. As we awaken each Organ through a specific sound, a positive Organ virtue is cultivated. Once all the Organs are awakened, they empower our moral character with high-minded virtues that manifest as goodwill.

Pure Mind correlates with the topmost energy point that crowns the top of the head. That point is known as Baihui, and when it is activated, we awaken benevolence. The cultivation of Pure Mind builds on the cultivation of Higher Mind. We use a specific technique to activate Baihui and we circulate Organ Qi through Baihui to integrate Pure Mind and Higher Mind. When the Crown is integrated with the Organ network, benevolence and goodwill spread throughout the body and we experience ourselves as blessed beings saturated with benevolence.

Spirit is associated with the Wuji Point, which is located in the area around the Lower Dantian. That point is a portal to an otherworldly realm that remains veiled until it is activated. When the Wuji point is activated, we enter Wuji and experience Perfect Peace. The meditation practice used to awaken the Organs and Higher Mind is called the Six Healing Sounds. The mediation practice to awaken Baihui and Pure Mind is called The Twelve Meridian Empowerment. And the meditation practice to awaken the Wuji Point and Spirit is called Huo Lu Gong (who-oh-loo-gong), which means Fire Furnace Practice.

Each meditation practice builds on the previous practice, and as we integrate the three practices, the benefits previously cultivated are amplified. As we awaken and integrate the energies of the Organs, we awaken goodwill. As we awaken and integrate the energy of Baihui, we awaken benevolence. As we awaken and integrate the energy produced by the Wuji Point, we awaken perfection. At each stage of our spiritual development, our virtue grows and becomes more robust. Practicing the sequence as it is presented is important. Do not skip ahead. Before detailing the instructions of the meditation practices, we will establish a deeper understanding of the bodymind connections. Once you grasp the structure of your bodymind as it relates to spiritual development, the mediations become vastly more meaningful and your progress gains momentum.

The Internal Organs

Individuals starting out on the spiritual journey sometimes presume that the more spiritually developed you are, the more detached you become from your negative emotions. They imagine the average person as someone who gets swept away by the river of emotions, and a spiritual master as an individual standing on the riverbank devoid of anger, fear, and worry. This idea is not exactly right. Spiritual masters experience negative emotions just like everyone else. But they possess the ability to transform those negative emotions into virtues.

Daoist sages were practical-minded, and they applied a thorough and systematic approach to their investigation of emotions. They observed the source of pain. If you stub your toe, your toe hurts. If you bump your elbow, your elbow hurts. If you bang your head, your head hurts. Physical pain is localized to the area that is injured. But what about emotional pain? When you feel anger, worry, or fear, where do you experience those emotions? We don't experience emotional pain in our big toe, elbow, or our head. Emotions originate somewhere within the cavity marked by our ribcage and extending down to our hips. We feel our emotions somewhere between the base of our neck and our lower abdomen.

Recall the last time you went on a first date with someone you really liked. Butterflies fluttered throughout your Small Intestine. Then, as you grew closer and intimate, you fell in love with this individual. You experienced joy and warmth in your Heart. Your whispered tender words that soothed your Lungs. You became excited at the prospect of a future together and your Liver burst with thunderous enthusiasm. But one night, you discovered your partner was cheating all along, and the relationship ended on a sour note. You felt betrayed. Where you once felt love, you now felt hate. Where you once felt tenderness, you now felt grief. Where you once felt enthusiasm, you now felt rage. In a matter of minutes, your positive emotions became negative emotions. Most of us have experienced some variation of this story. Most of us have been badly wounded by a relationship. If we pay careful attention to that experience, we observe that the emotional roller-coaster ride unfolds inside our torso. Daoist sages linked both positive and negative emotions to our Internal Organs. Daoist sages reasoned that emotions are so powerful that unless these forces were harnessed in a positive way, they could upend the spiritual journey. To avert this complication, they developed a method to transform negative emotions into positive virtues. This method involved meditating on the Internal Organs.

We live in an age of supermarkets that sell vacuum-packed, large-scale farmed chickens with empty cavities. Many of us have never cleaned out a whole chicken with our bare hands, but if you buy poultry from a small farm or a local butcher you are likely to find the organs intact. Once you open up the bird, you have to peel off the fascia, the thin rubbery layer of connective tissue that keeps the internal structures in place. As you clean out the bird, you would find a Heart, Lungs, a Liver, Kidneys, and a Spleen, as well as the Small and Large Intestines, Gallbladder, Urinary Bladder, and Stomach. Those same Internal Organs and Viscera exist inside the human body. They exist inside your body and before long you will develop a close relationship with them.

Daoist sages were intimately familiar with the Internal Organs. They made a distinction between the Internal Organs and the Viscera. The Internal Organs such as the Liver, Heart, Spleen, Lungs, and Kidneys were solid, while the Viscera such as the Gallbladder, Small Intestine, Stomach, Large Intestine, and Urinary Bladder were the hollow tubes that processed partially digested food and liquids and pushed out waste. They attributed the quality of Yin to the Internal Organs and Yang to the Viscera. They paired each Internal Organ with one of the Viscus.

The Lungs were paired with the Large Intestine, the Kidneys were paired with the Urinary Bladder, the Liver was paired with the Gallbladder, the Heart was paired with the Small Intestine, and the Spleen was paired with the Stomach. In total, there were five Internal Organs and five Viscera creating a system consisting of five Yin and Yang pairs. They added a sixth pair to the mix and this last pair was qualitatively different than the other five. The sixth Yin Organ was the Pericardium, the protective sac around the Heart, and the sixth Yang Organ was named San Jiao, which means the Triple Burner or the Triple Energizer.

San Jiao

San Jiao was mysteriously referred to as the Organ with a name but no form. But the meaning of this mystery is quickly revealed when you picture a bowl of fruit. You toss the bowl up in the air and the apples, peaches, and grapes fly off in different directions. If you swaddle the fruit with plastic wrap and toss the bowl, the fruit will hold together. What is the shape of the plastic wrap? The wrap has a name but no form. Replace the grapes with a large melon and the wrap conforms to the new shape. There is an internal structure within the human body that performs the same function as the plastic wrap: fascia. This connective tissue wraps around every internal structure including bones, nerves, blood vessels, muscles, tendons, and ligaments, as well as the Internal Organs and Viscera. Fascia literally keeps us from flying apart internally. The fascia in the trunk of the body is divided into three compartments. The upper compartment wraps around the Lungs and the Heart. The middle compartment extends from the diaphragm to the navel and includes the Spleen, Stomach, Liver, and Gallbladder. The lower compartment extends down from the navel to the pelvis, and includes the Kidneys, Urinary Bladder, and the Small and Large Intestines.

The three-fold division of the Organs and Viscera by fascia makes up San Jiao, the Triple Burner. San Jiao is also said to regulate the waterways—the extracellular fluids that flow between layers of fascia. In recent years, Western science has come to recognize fascia and extracellular fluid as a new organ—the largest in the body—called the interstitium. Broadly speaking, San Jiao can be associated with the interstitium. Narrowly speaking, San Jiao can be associated with the three-fold division of fascia between the Lungs and the Large Intestine.

Going forward, we will refer to the six pairs of Yin Internal Organs and Yang Viscera as the Six Organ Families. They are listed below:

The Six Organ Families	Yin Internal Organ	Yang Viscera
The Liver Family	Liver	Gallbladder
The Heart Family	Heart	Small Intestine
The Spleen Family	Spleen	Stomach
The Lung Family	Lungs	Large Intestine
The Kidney Family	Kidneys	Urinary Bladder
The San Jiao Family	Pericardium	San Jiao

Notice that each of the first five families is named after the Yin organ. Traditionally, the sixth family, San Jiao, is named after the Yang Viscus to distinguish this family from the other five. The reason for this distinction will become apparent when we explore the nature of each Organ Family in more depth. Additionally, we capitalize the name of the Internal Organs and Viscera to distinguish their spiritual function from their physiological function. And going forward, for the sake of simplicity, we will refer to both the Internal Organs and Viscera simply as the *Organs*.

Higher Mind and the Organ Network

Through direct experience, Daoist sages observed that each member of the Six Organ Families is associated with a positive emotional quality or virtue. When the Qi energy of the Organ was healthy and in a state of flow, the virtue of the Organ would arise naturally whenever needed. But if that energy was repressed, the positive emotion would transform into a negative emotion. The negative emotion could be directed inwardly at oneself, or it could be projected outwardly at someone else.

Let's concretize this model of emotional dynamics by considering the virtue and the two negative qualities associated with the Gallbladder. The virtue of the Gallbladder is *courage*. To have "gall" is to have the audacity to overcome a challenge through bold action that requires courage. The Gallbladder is associated with the urge to win. It is the part of us that is willing to face perilous uncertainty for the sake of victory. If you're in a potato sack race hopping around fiercely while focused on crossing the finish line first, you're drawing on your Gallbladder Qi. If your Gallbladder Qi is strong, you'll push hard and you won't give up, whatever happens.

We can personify a virtue by associating it with an archetype. Relating emotions to archetypes is a useful technique that humanizes and clarifies emotional dynamics. Someone who is courageous, audacious, and bold embodies the archetype of the Brave Warrior. The virtuous archetype of the Gallbladder is the Brave Warrior. Think of a courageous Coast Guard pilot who has participated in numerous rescue missions. Each mission, she faces perilous conditions that call for extreme courage. This pilot is a Brave Warrior. An entrepreneur who risks his life savings to start a new business resonates with the archetype as well.

The projection of courage into the world requires intention. We do not become a Brave Warrior unconsciously and reflexively. A daring and difficult choice has to be made to confront risk with temerity and fortitude. We can also choose to turn our back on courage. When a situation arises that calls for courage and we fall short of enacting the archetype of the Brave Warrior, the energy of the Gallbladder is repressed. Repressed Gallbladder energy does not disappear. It becomes negative energy that can manifest as *timidity* or *aggression*. Timidity is inwardly repressed courage. Aggression is the outward appearance of bravery but without the element of courage. It is false bravery. Both negative emotions are the shadow expressions of Gallbladder Qi.

Repressed Organ energies are also associated with negative archetypes. Timidity gives rise to the archetype of the Weakling and aggression to the Bully. The Brave Warrior, the Timid Weakling, and the Aggressive Bully are expressions of Gallbladder Qi and collectively they define the psychological domain of the Gallbladder. In the next chapter we will explore the qualities of each Organ in more detail. Our purpose now is to highlight the dynamics underlying the flow of Organ Qi. To solidify our understanding, we will consider the emotional qualities associated with the Lungs, which are markedly different than those of the Gallbladder.

A coworker lost her beloved cat over the weekend. She is sitting passively at her desk. Her posture is drooping forward. Her breathing is slightly labored. She is sniffling. You approach her.

"I am sorry to hear about your loss," you say.

"Thank you," she replies. There is a picture of her cat playing with a ball of yarn on her desk.

"Your cat was very cute," you say.

"She was adorable."

"What was her name?" you ask.

"Mildred," she replies.

"May Mildred's soul rest in peace."

"Thank you."

A week later, your coworker taps you on your shoulder and you turn around.

"I wanted to thank you for your sympathy. I was going through a rough patch, and you made me feel better. You are a Kind Soul."

The moral of this story is that kindness, the Organ Virtue of the Lungs, heals grief. The courage of the Gallbladder would not resonate with the grief of the Lungs. Trying to cheer up someone who is grieving with humor doesn't work either. Reasoning why they shouldn't be sad doesn't work. Berating them over their sadness doesn't work. The one virtue with the power to transform grief is kindness. And if you are feeling sad and practice kindness toward another person, your own grief will also be transformed. Kindness transforms grief into more kindness. The relationship between kindness and grief becomes self-evident once you experience their connection.

But kindness can be also repressed. Imagine that Mildred's owner is unwilling to receive your kindness. She rejects the kindness that you offered by scoffing at you. She suppresses the sadness she is feeling back into her Lungs repeatedly and her grief never heals. Over time, her Lungs become a storage bin of negativity and Lung Qi pathologies develop. Imagine that twelve years have passed, and she is still grieving Mildred. She is deeply depressed and still bemoaning the injustice of her loss. She has become fixated on a negative emotion and her Lungs are festering with grief. She has become the Gloomy Downer whose sadness overflows and colors every occasion. Just standing next to her by the water cooler you feel oppressed by her overbearing melancholy.

At the other extreme, we can imagine a person who lacks the ability to grieve altogether. They are desensitized to situations that call for grief. Imagine losing a household pet and feeling nothing. There is no sadness. No grief. No sense of loss. Just a black hole of numbness. This person knows they should be sad and pretends to grieve but feels nothing inside. This person embodies the archetype of the Shallow Griever. Although these two examples of avoiding grief are seemingly opposed, they share a commonality. Neither is capable of expressing or receiving genuine kindness. Both are examples of unhealthy Lung Qi.

When we repress an Organ Virtue repeatedly, that Organ becomes negatively charged and we are likely to become triggered by the positive expression of that energy. If our Lungs are negatively charged and we lack the capacity for kindness, for example, we become irritated by someone who is grieving and in need of the kindness that we are unable to express. Or, if our Gallbladder is negatively charged and we lack the capacity for courage, we become frustrated by someone who is in need of the encouragement that we are unable to express. When we are unable to express goodwill because an Organ Virtue is repressed, we generally express ill will. We can project ill will toward ourselves, an individual, a group, or the collective. In any event, repressed Organ Qi creates dissonance, separation, strife, and friction.

The Organs between our Lungs and our Large Intestine are teeming with virtues such as courage, kindness, enthusiasm, clarity, discernment, fairness, and caution, and repressed emotions such as timidity, grievance, arrogance, dissatisfaction, pessimism, anger, worry, disgust, and cruelty, among others. Virtuous archetypes such as the Brave Warrior, Comforter, Teacher, Nurturer, and Emperor, and repressed archetypes such as the Monster, Dictator, Disruptor, and Lost Soul arise from the condition of our Organs. The Organ network, and the emotional realm it embodies, represents the physiological aspect of Higher Mind.

The Central Role of the Heart

Daoist sages also observed that the Heart plays a central role in relation to all the other Organs. Specifically, all the emotions filter through the Heart as we express them in the world. They associated the Heart with the archetype of the Emperor. The Heart had the final say in matters of Higher Mind and its virtue of honor was essential for our overall emotional well-being.

The metaphor of a piano can help us visualize the relationship between Higher Mind and the twelve Organs. In this example, the twelve notes that constitute the keys of an octave represent the twelve Organs. When you strike a key, the sound can be well-tuned and consonant or out of tune and dissonant. Similarly, the emotional "tone" struck by an Organ can be well-tuned or out of tune. A well-tuned Gallbladder conveys courage while an out of tune Gallbladder conveys repressed courage in the form of timidity or aggression.

Higher Mind represents the entire keyboard with the Heart representing C major. As the melody of life plays out, eventually the dissonant notes will strike a strident sound. If you were listening to a melody on a piano with just one defective key, would you be able to ignore the dissonant note? It is likely that your attention would be drawn to the dissonant note that would drown out all the others. Similarly, awareness is drawn to the repressed Organs, qualities that require fine-tuning and integration. If the Gallbladder is a dissonant note on your "piano," the themes of timidity and aggression will play out repeatedly in your life. You will attract Weaklings and Bullies until you manage to integrate Gallbladder Qi, express authentic courage, and embody the archetype of the Brave Warrior.

The school of hard knocks is the long-winded way to tune our pianos. There is a shorter and more efficient method to integrate and harmonize the Organ Virtues and balance Higher Mind. Through meditation, we can transform our repressed emotional qualities into Organ Virtues. Instead of suffering through endless drama that reflects our dissonance, we can cultivate Higher Mind and manifest the capacity for goodwill. The meditation that we practice to cultivate Higher Mind is called the Six Healing Sounds. As you become proficient at this practice, you awaken an Organ, release the repressed Organ Qi trapped within, and empower the Organ Virtue. As a result, you cultivate Higher Mind and build moral character in the process.

Pure Mind and Baihui

Picture a knight in shining armor. He fights for justice. He is brave and loyal. He embodies courage and kindness. He is admired for his moral character and goodwill. His Organs are healthy and radiate positive energy. His Higher Mind is refined. He is standing beside a holy woman. She embodies moral character as well, but she emanates an additional quality that he lacks. In her presence, we experience benevolence. She sits silently and puts her hands together to pray and she exudes an aura of sacredness. Even the gallant knight recognizes her divinity and bows at her feet for her blessing.

Sacredness includes morality but also transcends it. Benevolence includes goodwill but also transcends it. But what is sacredness and from where does it arise?

Picture a group of refugees huddled in a tent. They are scared, hungry, and cold. At mealtime, they are given a miserly plate of food. A toddler is crying because she is still hungry. A stranger approaches the girl's mother and hands her his food without speaking a word. The mother takes the food and gives it to the girl who eats it quietly. Across the tent, the girl's grandfather witnesses the gracious act and his eyes well up with tears. These are not tears of sadness. Saintly acts of sacrifice inspire sacred tears. A man jumps into a river to save a boy that has fallen in. Perhaps he saves the boy. Perhaps he dies trying to save the boy. Either way, this sacrificial act also inspires sacred tears.

Imagine now that you are in the presence of the Divine Mother in whatever symbolic form she manifests to you. Divine Mother is the archetype associated with the sacrificial aspect of compassion. She is crying inconsolably, and her tears are flowing like rivers and flooding the ground.

You place your hand gingerly on her shoulder and ask, "Divine Mother, are you sad?"

"No, my child," she replies, still sobbing.

"Are you in pain?"

"No, my child," she replies.

"Then why are you crying inconsolably?"

"These are divine tears. Every benevolent act performed by a human is worthy of a tear."

Selfless acts of sacrifice create the quality of reverence that prompts sacred tears. Benevolence prompts sacred tears. When you act benevolently, Divine Mother sheds a tear for you. Imagine that you are in that relationship we mentioned previously that ends badly. You can project ill will or even malevolence at your former partner. That is the typical emotional arc that follows a breakup. But what if instead of projecting negativity you pray for the well-being and growth of your former partner? Divine Mother would shed a tear. If you pray for the healing and well-being of your enemy, she will shed another tear. What if you prayed for the healing and well-being of all sentient beings? Her tears would flood the world.

The tears of Divine Mother are prompted by benevolence, and energetically benevolence is associated with a specific energy point called Baihui. Baihui literally means "hundred meetings" or "the place where one hundred converge into one." It is located at the top of the head. Baihui is the point where Heaven Qi meets Human Qi. The "hundred meetings" refers to the many celestial energies that funnel into our energy body. At Baihui, we draw in the energy of the sun, moon, planets, and stars. The one hundred also refers to our personal energies that spout from us and flow into the sky. Baihui processes communication between Heaven and Human continuously. Once awakened, Baihui generates the feeling of sacredness and inspires benevolence. Baihui is the abode of Pure Mind.

When we witness benevolence, our Baihui is activated, and we are filled with the feeling of reverence. When we cultivate Baihui through meditation practice, we can access that quality more readily. When Baihui is wide open and receptive, we can invoke the feeling of sacredness at will and evoke the presence of benevolence through our mere presence. We feel as though Divine Mother is our constant companion.

When Baihui is integrated with the Heart, Higher Mind and Pure Mind come into alignment. As the Organ Virtues blend with benevolence, we develop the power to bless. A blessing is the integration of goodwill and benevolence. A blessing fuses Heart Qi and Baihui Qi. When Pure Mind is awakened and refined, our inner life is infused with the divine power to bless. Imagine a father blessing his beloved daughter on her wedding day. The space around them is teeming with the quality of sacredness. Energetically, his Heart Qi and Baihui Qi are activated. Poetically, the Emperor is wearing his Crown. If you were to paint the scene, you might be inspired to draw a nimbus around the father's head. And if the daughter's Heart and Baihui are open to her father's blessing, we could draw a nimbus around her head as well.

When Baihui Qi is integrated with Organ Qi, the Organ Virtues are endowed with benevolence, and we develop the capacity for magnificent acts of goodness in the face of evil. Imagine a tyrannical regime ruled by a malevolent despot. The people are controlled by fear. The willingness to confront this regime requires more than just courage. It requires sacrificial courage. Sacrificial courage is qualitatively different than the courage required to start a new business. Courage is not enough to confront malevolence. Benevolent courage is required. When a Brave Warrior is inspired by Baihui Qi, they are transformed into a Divine Warrior who is prepared to sacrifice themselves to battle evil.

The meditation we practice to awaken Baihui and to integrate Baihui with the Organ Virtues is called the Twelve Meridian Empowerment. As you become proficient at this practice, you awaken your capacity for benevolence and integrate that quality with the Organs. As a result, you cultivate Pure Mind and empower your moral character with divine qualities.

Spirit and the Wuji Point

The notion that Spirit is associated with an energy point located in the area of the navel sounds odd at first. After all, Spirit represents an otherworldly aspect of our identity. If you were searching for a gateway to Spirit inside the body, you might think to look elsewhere. But Daoist sages realized that the safest and most direct route to Spirit runs though the Wuji Point. The Wuji Point is a special energy point, and it has to be activated by a specific method detailed in chapter 6. Once you awaken the Wuji Point and experience the realm of Spirit, you realize right away that you are entering a different kind of existential space.

The quality of the energy arising from the Wuji Point feels qualitatively different than Organ Qi or even Baihui Qi. Once the Wuji Point is activated, something magical happens. You feel as though a portal to another dimension opens, and a unique form of energy flows into your body. Usually, when we circulate energy, we feel a current of Qi moving along a path through the physical body. We might even be able to project energy outside the body, or absorb energy from another object, like a tree or a flower, into the body. The quality of Spirit is an altogether different experience. It is not an energy that we circulate. As we awaken Spirit, it feels as though we are entering another world. Or perhaps this other world enters us. It is hard to tell the difference between the two because the energy of Spirit erases division lines and boundaries.

The Wuji Point acts as a veil that separates Wuji from duality. Most of our lives, we are bound to the realm of duality, which is subject to the laws of Yin and Yang. Our physiology is constantly trying to maintain homeostasis. Our minds are constantly choosing between likes and dislikes, right and wrong, and good and evil. We prioritize, rank, and evaluate. We desire and reject. The realm of duality is a world of constant movement, contrast, and choice. Being in a state of Oneness extinguishes duality. Experiencing the unified wholeness of Spirit is a profound experience.

Imagine that you are in a cloud. What do you see? Is the cloud small or big? You can't tell. Are you three hundred feet above ground or thirty thousand feet above ground? You can't tell. Are you facing east or west? You can't tell. You can open your eyes or close them, and it does not make a difference. Inside a thick cloud, your senses, which divide the world into a multitude of categories, become useless. As Spirit permeates our being, we feel as though we are shrouded in a Primordial Cloud. This Primordial Cloud is timeless and spaceless. It dissolves boundaries and opens into a wondrous spaciousness that is boundless. As our sense of separation dissolves, our body sense dissolves. Our identity dissolves. Our thoughts and feelings dissolve. We disappear as a solitary human being and emerge as an endless expanse of well-being.

Usually, when we sit for meditation, thoughts come and go. But as we abide in the Primordial Cloud, there are no stray thoughts. When you are not hungry you don't think of food. When you are not cold, you don't think of warmth. When you are not worried, your mind doesn't race around looking for solutions to problems. Imagine being very thirsty and someone hands you a glass of water. The moment your desire for water is extinguished, there is a feeling of deep satisfaction. Being inside the Primordial Cloud is like capturing that moment and spreading it to all unmet desires. The extinction of desire that arises as we settle into unified Oneness is peace. It is perfection. Abiding as Spirit in Wuji is Perfect Peace.

A sense of deep well-being characterizes the Oneness of Spirit. The sensation is so profoundly satisfying and soothing that all defenses drop. The ego is extinguished. Psychological drives are extinguished. Thoughts are extinguished. Without thoughts, suffering disappears. Without sensations, pain disappears. Without an identity, our sense of separateness disappears.

Within the Primordial Cloud, the tributaries of mind merge into the ocean of Spirit, and our Original Self arises. Wuji is the answer to the koans, *What is your original name? What is your original face?* Your original name is Spirit. Your original face is Perfect Peace. Perfect Peace is who you become when you abide as Spirit. My Master, Xiao Yao, referred to the perfection of Wuji as the *Hunyuan State.* "Hunyuan means Primordial. It is what came before Yin and Yang," he explained. "This way of being defines our original unified state. It is the self-accomplished state. There is nothing to add or remove to make Hunyuan more perfect than it is. In the Hunyuan State you are perfect as you are."

Every human being yearns to feel at home and to experience endless peace. This desire is the mother of all desires. You earn a million dollars, and you are satisfied for a short while before you want to make another million. A promotion satisfies your ambition only for a short while before you hunger for more. A delicious meal satisfies your appetite for a short while, but tomorrow you'll wake up hungry again. The postnatal realm, the world of duality, is a never-ending roller-coaster ride. Momentary periods of calm are punctuated by turmoil. The incessant drama of life exhausts the psyche. The exhausted psyche yearns for peace. Like a bird flying over a wide ocean, we grow tired and want to find a place to rest. Abiding as Spirit is the antidote to the existential suffering that arises from the travails of duality. Abiding as Spirit, we finally come home. We finally find peace.

When we awaken as Spirit and reengage the world, we experience ourselves differently. Our body no longer feels dense and heavy. We no longer perceive ourselves as a covering of skin holding together flesh, blood, and bones. We experience ourselves as beings of light. The feeling of spaciousness remains in the foreground of awareness. Our organs feel like fields of swirling energy. Our Dantians feel like whirling spheres of energy. Our fingers feel like beams of energy. The opacity of the physical body becomes a translucent matrix of energy.

As we walk down the street, the world arises within our Oneness. The trees and stars and the people whom we love arise in the spaciousness of Spirit. Wuji becomes the central focus of awareness and permeates our moment-to-moment interactions. You shake hands with another person and experience two energy currents coming together. You admire a sunset and experience the energy swirls of a Van Gogh sky. The entire cosmos rises and sets as a composition of energy in the spaciousness of awareness, and a sense of perfection pervades the world, imperfect though it may be.

Spirit expresses the quality of Wu Wei—unified doing through nondoing. When you abide as Spirit in the material world, you find yourself at the right place at the right time. You avoid the wrong place at the wrong time. You attract the right people and avoid the wrong people. You take the right action and speak the right words. A sense of coherence pervades the disorder streaming through your life. Spirit provokes synchronicities. Meaningful patterns and relationships mediated by Spirit arise effortlessly. Your life orchestrates a meaningful adventure that actualizes the full potential of your being.

The spaciousness of Spirit enhances the emotions that we feel. We experience our emotions in vivid colors. We experience sadness, kindness, courage, and anger, and all other emotions within the spaciousness of Spirit. Any emotional turmoil that we experience self-organizes into deeper understanding. Spirit transforms pandemonium into peace.

As we awaken as Spirit, we identify with the peaceful spaciousness that envelops our experience of the world. Our social identities become secondary. We are no longer a truck driver or a teacher, we are no longer a man or a woman, we are no longer bound to race, religion, or gender. We identify primarily as Spirit. We realize our Oneness and perceive the

Oneness in all other human beings. We look another human in the eyes and recognize their Spirit. A Spirit-identified being embodies the deep desire to end the suffering of all the beings who are dissociated from the Primordial Realm. A deep desire emerges to draw others into the experience of Perfect Peace.

When we encounter someone who embodies peacefulness, holiness, and a high moral character, we experience serenity. The sense of peace they radiate stills our mind. The benevolence they radiate is a humbling blessing. The sense of integrity they embody inspires us to goodness. In their presence many of the problems we experience fall away. The presence of a human being that has traveled The Way of Virtue endows our lives with a sense of coherence. Through their being, we get a sneak preview of the possibilities inherent in our own lives. The presence of a spiritual master is a transmission that inspires us to become a more complete version of ourselves.

My master, Xiao Yao, was benevolent and overflowed with goodwill. Even though he was orphaned at a young age, lost his privileged position as the abbot of his monastery during the Cultural Revolution, and lived in abject poverty doing menial work well into in his eighties, he never once expressed the slightest speck of negativity. I never heard him say anything negative about anyone. I never heard him wish anyone ill. I never heard him complain about anything. I never heard him disrespect or mock another human being, even in private. He was always positive and happy and radiated a deep sense of peace. His bravery was legend as was his kindness. He was willing to help anyone, anytime, without expecting anything in return. His mind was perfectly peaceful, and his presence was a beautiful melody that enchanted. His remarkable character was the reflection of the spiritual practices that he was taught by his master. These are the practices that he taught me and that I will be sharing with you. The practices were developed by spiritual geniuses and refined by a long line of spiritual masters. They worked for Xiao Yao, they worked for me, and they will work for you as well.

The three mediation practices presented over the next three chapters define The Way of Virtue. The first practice, the Six Healing Sounds, awakens and empowers Higher Mind and cultivates goodwill and the Organ Virtues. The second practice, The Twelve Meridian Empowerment, awakens and empowers Pure Mind and cultivates the virtue of benevolence. The third practice, Huo Lu Gong, awakens and empowers Spirit and cultivates the virtue of Perfect Peace.

The table below summarizes the relationship between the three practices and the virtues they awaken.

Practice	Cultivation of Mind	The Way of Virtue
Six Healing Sounds	Higher Mind	Organ Virtues
Twelve Meridian Empowerment	Pure Mind	Benevolence
Huo Lu Gong	Spirit	Perfect Peace

Exercise 11: Wogu—Protecting Against Negativity

Xiao Yao was good, but he was not naive. He understood that human beings can be vicious and that their negativity can adversely influence a spiritual practitioner. He taught me two simple practices to protect myself from the negativity of other people. The first is a hand gesture, or mudra, that we can use to protect ourselves from the negativity generated by another person. Hand gestures operate on the principle that your hand represents your energy field and that the gestures that you create with your hand transform your energy field. The protective hand gesture Xiao Yao taught me is called Wogu. Wo means "hold" and Gu means "firm." By doing Wogu you concentrate the outer layer of your Qi field, known as Guardian Qi, around your body without signaling aggression. Wogu is a deflector shield that insulates you from negativity. If someone is projecting negativity toward us and we practice Wogu, the energy bounces back at them. The next time your boss scolds you, practice Wogu. The negative energy will bounce back at them, and they will tire quickly and stop.

Figure 4.1: Wogu Hand Gesture

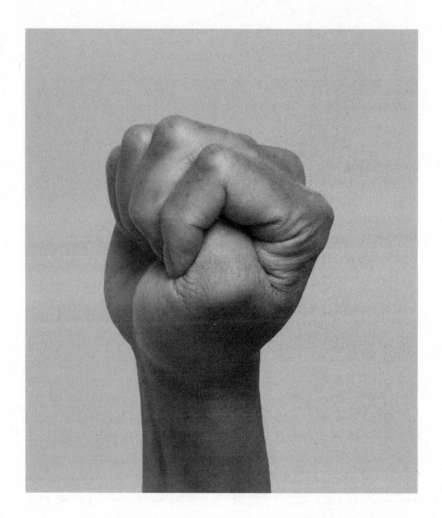

Sometimes, we can't use our hands to form a hand gesture. You may be carrying something or it may be socially inappropriate. In those instances, you can create Wogu by clamping your toes.

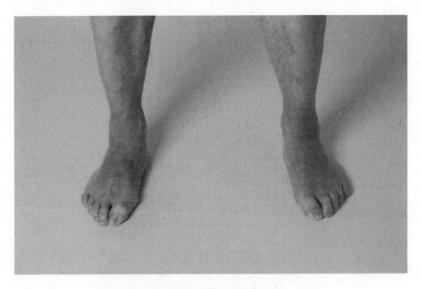

Figure 4.2: Clamping Toes

1. Make loose fists and wrap your fingers around your thumbs as indicated in the image above. If you are not able to do Wogu, perhaps you are holding papers or sitting in close proximity to the person projecting the negativity, clamp your toes on the ground. The effect is the same.

2. Maintain either position until the negativity abates.

Exercise 12: Awaken Your Inner Smile

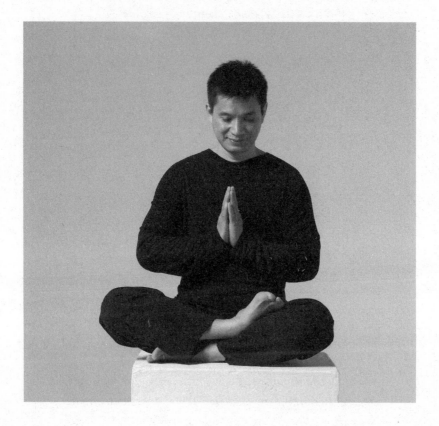

Figure 4.3: Buddha Smiling

Picture the most beautiful face you have ever seen. It is youthful and the symmetry harmonizes the features. The skin is tight. The complexion is clear. Sixty years from now, that face will be eighty years old. Will people still use the word "beautiful" to describe that face? Maybe . . . Some faces remain beautiful despite the wrinkles. What makes a face perpetually beautiful is the smiling energy it radiates. Have you ever noticed the quality of a smile? A dour face will force a smile and as soon as it turns away that dour look will return and erase that smile quickly. You can't fake a genuine smile. When you smile, really smile, you radiate well-being that arises from within. A real smile is infectious and spreads positive energy.

You will often see statues or paintings of Buddha depicted with a smile. Some of his smiles are subtle and others depict laughter. Buddha's inner radiance and his smile are inseparable from his virtues. When you cultivate your own Buddha smile, you open up space for benevolence and goodwill to arise.

My master, Xiao Yao, had a memorable smile that still warms my heart when I recall it. He encouraged me to practice smiling often. Gradually, I noticed that smiling became easier and more natural. After some time, the joyful energy I was cultivating in my meditations flowed effortlessly to my face. Eventually, the smiling energy became a constant feature. The feeling of well-being that I experienced inwardly overflowed into my social interactions, and sharing that energy sweetens my day.

Smiling can be practiced anytime, anywhere: before a meditation, after a meditation, in the morning when you wake up, while you are interacting with other people. Practice inner smiling until a subtle smile becomes effortless and a natural feature of your face.

1. Imagine a spiritual teacher, a saint, a holy person from any tradition (like Buddha), or the person who loves you the most smiling at you. You can also picture a three-year-old version of yourself smiling at you. Smiles are contagious. Let their smile activate your smile.

2. Feel the smiling energy rise up from your Lower Dantian like a thousand tiny bubbles stirring every cell in your body to smile. Feel the bubbles rise to your face and smile. Practice smiling until your smile becomes your constant companion.

Wogu and smiling are complementary practices. Wogu dispels negativity and a smile creates positivity. Practice Wogu while you smile inwardly. Feeling positive energy flowing to your lips and face will help scatter the negativity. On your journey to Spirit, these practices will serve you well.

Part 2

THE JOURNEY TO SPIRIT

5

The Six Healing Sounds

Locating Your Organs

Imagine you are sitting in front of a piano with your foot on the damper pedal. Next to you is an opera singer. She sings a note. After she stops, you can hear piano strings sounding that same note. No one touched the key and yet the vibration of her voice caused the strings to vibrate. The ability to use sound vibration to activate another object at a distance is called resonance. Resonance can be used to activate an Organ. Resonance can be used to release the repressed energy of an Organ. And resonance can be used to empower an Organ Virtue.

Daoist sages discovered resonant sounds that activate the Six Organ Families. They discovered that a specific sound can be used to activate an Organ Pair. For example, the Lungs and Large Intestine both vibrate to the same resonance. That's like signing a particular note that resonates with two piano strings. Chant another sound and another Organ Pair begins to vibrate. Only six resonant sounds are needed to activate the Six Organ Families.

Getting these sounds just right requires experimentation. We have different voices. The shapes of our mouths and lips differ. Our body structures differ. If the resonance of an Organ sound is off by just a little, your Organs won't vibrate properly, no matter how long you chant. So how do you determine the right resonance for you?

Daoist sages solved this problem when they discovered that each one of the six sounds that resonate with an Organ Pair also resonates with one of the sense organs on our face. When the Lung Family sound resonates, for example, our Nose also vibrates. The Lung sound vibrates the Nose, Lungs, and Large Intestine. Since it is easier to vibrate the Nose than it is to vibrate the Lungs and Large Intestine, they reasoned that the most direct way to fine-tune the Lung sound was to chant the sound until our Nose vibrated most strongly, and then to direct that same resonance to the Lungs and Large Intestine.

The connection between the Nose and the Lungs makes intuitive sense since the air we inhale though our nostrils fills our Lungs. But what qualifies the Nose for membership in the Lung Family is the shared resonance. A similar relationship exists between the Eyes and the Liver Family, the Tongue and the Heart Family, the Mouth and Lips and the Spleen Family, the Ears and the Kidney Family, and the entire Face and the San Jiao Family. We begin chanting the six Organ sounds, which are known as the Six Healing Sounds, by fine-tuning the resonance so that it vibrates its related sense Organ. This is like musicians tuning their instruments before their performance.

If you rub your hands vigorously and place your palms a few inches apart, you can feel the Qi energy between them vibrating. We can't rub our Stomach the way we rub our palms, but we can use the Spleen Healing Sound to activate our Mouth and Lips and then direct that vibration to the Stomach. If we repeat the chant several times, we experience our Stomach vibrating its own Qi energy: Stomach Qi. By mastering the Six Healing Sounds, which are described in the coming pages, we can awaken our Organs in a matter of minutes. This simple technique is the basis for the Six Healing Sounds Meditation.

Traditionally, the Yin Organ is called the mother of an Organ Family, the Yang Organ is called the father, and the sense Organ is called the child. The mothers of the Ears are the Kidneys, the father of the Ears is the Urinary Bladder. Or we can say that the Ears are the children of the Kidney Family.

The table below depicts family relations between the Organs:

Six Organ Families	Mother	Father	Child
Liver Family	Liver	Gallbladder	Eyes
Heart Family	Heart	Small Intestine	Tongue
Spleen Family	Spleen	Stomach	Mouth and Lips
Lung Family	Lungs	Large Intestine	Nose
Kidney Family	Kidneys	Urinary Bladder	Ears
San Jiao Family	Pericardium	San Jiao	Face

In the section that follows, we awaken the Six Healing Sounds, one at a time. We begin by resonating with the Child, then the Mother, and then the Father. Once you experience all three vibrating, you can repeat the chant and keep the entire family resonating. While all the sounds are relatively simple, I find that the Spleen Family Sound, which resonates with the Mouth and Lips, is the easiest for most people to experience. You may wish to skip ahead and start with that sound to settle into the process. Once you can resonate with the Spleen Family Sound, please return to the sequence presented below. The sequence begins with the Liver sound.

Exercise 13: Awaken Your Liver Family

Liver Family

- Name of Chant: Xu
- Healing Sound: *Shewww . . .*
- Mother: Liver
- Father: Gallbladder
- Children: Eyes

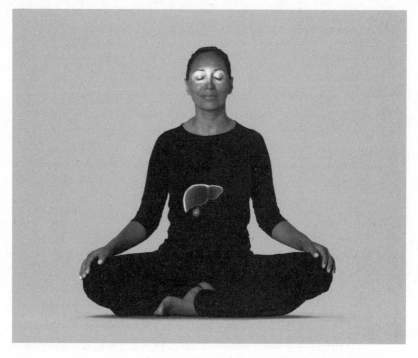

Figure 5.1: Liver, Gallbladder, and Eyes

Exercise Summary

If you tap your ribs on the right side and then on the left side, you will notice that the tapping sound each side makes is different. The sensation between both sides feels different. The right side feels solid while the left side feels hollow. The reason for that difference is that the Liver is situated on the right side. The Liver is about the size of a football and weighs around three pounds. The Gallbladder is a pear-shaped organ between three and six inches long located under the Liver. The Eyes are the children of the Liver Family.

Adopt the natural sitting position. Proper spinal alignment and a relaxed ribcage are essential to finding the right resonance. The Liver Family Chant is named Xu, pronounced *shew.* The healing sound of Xu is pronounced *shewww* . . . The healing sound is intoned like the word *shoe* with the tail end trailing until you run out of air. Chant naturally. Do not strain. As you resonate Xu, you will feel your upper palate vibrate and the vibration will extend upward to your Eyes. Chant Xu three or more times until you feel your Eyes vibrating. Take as much time as feels appropriate in between chants.

Once both Eyes are vibrating, chant Xu and direct the resonance to your Liver. Take as much time as feels appropriate in between chants. Feel the entire Liver vibrate, front and back, top and bottom, and the center. Once you feel the Eyes and the Liver vibrating, direct the healing sound to the Gallbladder and repeat the process. Feel the three members of the Liver Family vibrate as you chant Xu. Continue to feel the vibration after the chanting ends.

Exercise Instruction

The formal instructions for this exercise are detailed below.

1. Adopt Natural Sitting Posture and close your eyes gently.

2. Practice Taiji Breathing for three cycles until your mind is calm.

3. Become aware of your Eyes. Chant Xu, *shewww* . . . Feel the healing sound vibrate your Eyes. Repeat three times or more.

4. Become aware of your Liver. Chant Xu, *shewww* . . . Feel the healing sound vibrate your Liver. Repeat three times or more.

5. Become aware of your Gallbladder. Chant Xu, *shewww* . . . Feel the healing sound vibrate your Gallbladder. Repeat three times or more.

6. Become aware of your Liver Family. Chant Xu, *shewww* . . . Feel the healing sound vibrate your Eyes, Liver, and Gallbladder. Repeat three times or more.

7. Continue to feel the vibration after the chanting ends.

8. Nourish your Eyes, Liver, and Gallbladder. *I am in Qi; Qi is in me.*

Exercise 14: Awaken Your Heart Family

Heart Family

- Name of Chant: Ha
- Healing Sound: *Haaaaa . . .*
- Mother: Heart
- Father: Small Intestine
- Child: Tongue

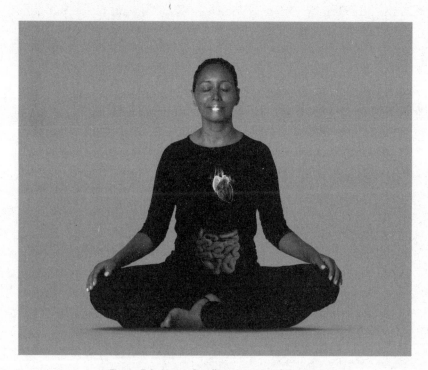

Figure 5.2: Heart, Small Intestine, and Tongue

Exercise Summary

The second healing sound in the series is the Heart Family Chant, Ha. The Organ Pair known as the Heart Family is made up of the Heart and Small Intestine. The Heart is the size of a fist and shaped like a lotus. It rests above the diaphragm in front of the fifth thoracic vertebra. The Heart is surrounded by the Pericardium, covered by the left Lung, and protected by the sternum. The Small Intestine is over twenty feet long and coiled in the lower abdominal cavity. It extends from the Stomach to the Large Intestine, which frames it.

The Tongue is the child of the Heart Family. The mother of the Tongue is the Heart, and the father of the tongue is the Small Intestine. Allow your Tongue to relax. Do not contact the roof of your mouth. Allow the weight of your Tongue to rest on the *root* of the Tongue. Let go of all the tension in your tongue. Usually, our Tongue is in perpetual motion so relaxing the Tongue may be a new experience. Once the Tongue is relaxed, really relaxed, chant Ha, *haaaaa* . . . Feel the healing sound vibrate your tongue.

Experiment until you hone in on the strongest frequency and then direct Ha to your Heart. Feel your Heart vibrate. Chant Ha several times. Direct Ha to your Small Intestine. Feel your Small Intestine vibrate. Then Chant Ha and feel the entire Heart Family vibrate. Continue to feel the vibration after the chanting ends.

Exercise Instruction

The formal instructions for this exercise are detailed below.

1. Adopt Natural Sitting Posture and close your eyes gently.

2. Practice Taiji Breathing for three cycles until your mind is calm.

3. Become aware of your Tongue. Chant Ha, *haaaaa* . . . Feel the healing sound vibrate your Tongue. Repeat three times or more.

4. Become aware of your Heart. Chant Ha, *haaaaa* . . . Feel the healing sound vibrate your Heart. Repeat three times or more.

5. Become aware of your Small Intestine. Chant Ha, *haaaaa* . . . Feel the healing sound vibrate your Small Intestine. Repeat three times or more.

6. Become aware of your Heart Family. Chant Ha, *haaaaa* . . . Feel the healing sound vibrate your Tongue, Heart, and Small Intestine. Repeat three times or more.

7. Continue to feel the vibration after the chanting ends.

8. Nourish your Tongue, Heart, and Small Intestine. *I am in Qi; Qi is in me.*

Exercise 15: Awaken Your Spleen Family

Spleen Family

- Name of Chant: Hu
- Healing Sound: *Whoooo* . . .
- Mother: Spleen
- Father: Stomach
- Children: Mouth and Lips

Exercise Summary

The third healing sound in the series is the Spleen Family Chant, Hu, pronounced *who*. The Organ Pair known as the Spleen Family is made up of the Spleen and the Stomach. The Spleen is located in the upper left part of the abdomen behind your ribs and the Stomach and beneath the diaphragm. It is about five inches long, three inches wide, and one and a half inches thick. It is shaped like a concave shell. The Stomach begins at

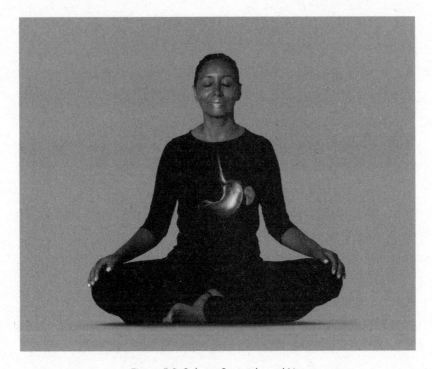

Figure 5.3: Spleen, Stomach, and Lips

the end of the esophagus and extends into the abdominal cavity, where it connects to the Small Intestine. It lies on the left side of the upper abdomen. It is about a foot long and six inches across.

The Mouth and Lips are the children of the Spleen Family. The mother of the Mouth and Lips is the Spleen, and the father of the Mouth and Lips is the Stomach.

Relax your cheeks and chant Hu, *whoooo* . . . Feel the healing sound vibrate the walls of your Mouth and Lips. When you feel your Mouth and Lips most strongly, you have discovered your resonance of Hu. Direct Hu to your Spleen. Feel your Spleen vibrate. Direct Hu to your Stomach. Feel your Stomach vibrate. Feel the entire Spleen Family vibrate as you chant Hu. Continue to feel the vibration after the chanting ends.

Exercise Instruction

The formal instructions for this exercise are detailed below.

1. Adopt Natural Sitting Posture and close your eyes gently.

2. Practice Taiji Breathing for three cycles until your mind is calm.

3. Become aware of your Mouth and Lips. Chant Hu, *whoooo* . . . Feel the healing sound vibrate your Mouth and Lips. Repeat three times or more.

4. Become aware of your Spleen. Chant Hu, *whoooo* . . . Feel the healing sound vibrate your Spleen. Repeat three times or more.

5. Become aware of your Stomach. Chant Hu, *whoooo* . . . Feel the healing sound vibrate your Stomach. Repeat three times or more.

6. Become aware of your Spleen Family. Chant Hu, *whoooo* . . . Feel the healing sound vibrate your Mouth and Lips, Spleen, and Stomach. Repeat three times or more.

7. Continue to feel the vibration after the chanting ends.

8. Nourish your Mouth and Lips, Spleen, and Stomach. *I am in Qi; Qi is in me.*

Exercise 16: Awaken Your Lung Family

Lung Family

- Name of Chant: Si
- Healing sound: *Szzzzzz* . . .
- Mother: Lungs
- Father: Large Intestine
- Child: Nose

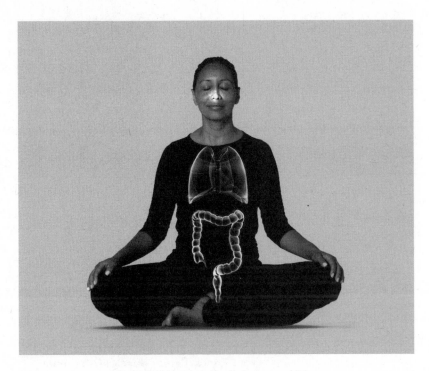

Figure 5.4: Lungs, Large Intestine, and Nose

Exercise Summary

The fourth healing sound in the series is the Lung chant, Si, pronounced like *sir* without the "r." The Organ Pair known as the Lungs is made up of the Lungs and the Large Intestine. The Lungs are spongy Organs located in the chest cavity on both sides of the sternum. They extend from the collar bone to the sixth rib on the front and reach down to the tenth rib in the back.

The Large Intestine is about five feet long and three inches in diameter. It frames the small intestine and empties out into the rectum.

The Nose is the child of the Lung Family. The mother of the Nose is the Lungs, and the father of the nose is the Large Intestine. The Lung chant Si is a droning sound pronounced, *szzzzzz* . . . Make an "s" sound followed by a buzzing "z" sound. This healing sounds like a buzzsaw. The vibration is focused on the front of your upper palate and from there it rises to your nose. Feel your Nose vibrate. When your Nose is vibrating most strongly, you have discovered Si. Direct the vibration to the Lungs. Feel your Lungs vibrate, *szzzzzz* . . . Direct Si to the Large Intestine. Feel the Large Intestine vibrate. Feel the entire Lung Family vibrate as you chant Si. Continue to feel the vibration after the chanting ends.

Exercise Instruction

The formal instructions for this exercise are detailed below.

1. Adopt Natural Sitting Posture and close your eyes gently.

2. Practice Taiji Breathing for three cycles until your mind is calm.

3. Become aware of your Nose. Chant Si, *szzzzz* . . . Feel the healing sound vibrate your Nose. Repeat three times or more.

4. Become aware of your Lungs. Chant Si, *szzzzz* . . . Feel the healing sound vibrate your Lungs. Repeat three times or more.

5. Become aware of your Large Intestine. Chant Si, *szzzzz* . . . Feel the healing sound vibrate your Large Intestine. Repeat three times or more.

6. Become aware of your Lung Family. Chant Si, *szzzzz* . . . Feel the healing sound vibrate your Nose, Lungs, and Large Intestine. Repeat three times or more.

7. Continue to feel the vibration after the chanting ends.

8. Nourish your Nose, Lungs, and Large Intestine. *I am in Qi; Qi is in me.*

Exercise 17: Awaken Your Kidney Family

Kidney Family

- Chant: Chui
- Healing sound: *Chuwee . . .*
- Mother: Kidneys
- Father: Urinary Bladder
- Children: Ears

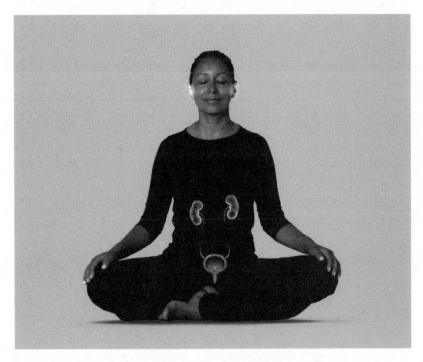

Figure 5.5: Kidneys, Urinary Bladder, and Ears

Exercise Summary

The fifth healing sound in the series is the Kidney Family Chant, Chui, pronounced *chewy*. The Organ Pair known as the Kidneys is made up of the Kidneys and the Urinary Bladder. The Kidneys are kidney bean–shaped Organs around five inches long. They extend below the ribs along the spine. The left Kidney is slightly higher than the right Kidney due to the position of the liver on the right side of the body.

The Urinary Bladder is attached by ligaments to the pelvic bones. It spans approximately twelve inches. When it is full, it extends into the lower abdominal cavity.

The Ears are the children of the Kidneys. The mothers of the Ears are the Kidneys and the father of the Ears is the Urinary Bladder. The Kidney healing sound is pronounced, *chuwee* . . . The sound begins with your lips puckered as you say, *chew*. Then your mouth stretches to the sides as you say *weeeee* . . . As you say *weeeee* . . . feel the vibration stretch across your face and extend all the way to your Ears. Feel the vibration activating the small inner bones as well as the cranial bones surrounding your ears. You may feel the vibration in one ear more distinctly at first. Modulate the chant until both ears are vibrating equally. Then direct the chant Chui to the Kidneys. Feel both Kidneys vibrate. Direct the chant Chui to the Urinary Bladder. Feel the Urinary Bladder vibrate, *chueee* . . . Feel the Kidney Organ Family vibrate as you chant Chui. Continue to feel the vibration after the chanting ends.

Exercise Instruction

The formal instructions for this exercise are detailed below.

1. Adopt Natural Sitting Posture and close your eyes gently.

2. Practice Taiji Breathing for three cycles until your mind is calm.

3. Become aware of your Ears. Chant Chui, *chuwee* . . . Feel the healing sound vibrate your Ears. Repeat three times or more.

4. Become aware of your Kidneys. Chant Chui, *chuwee . . .* Feel the healing sound vibrate your Kidneys. Repeat three times or more.

5. Become aware of your Urinary Bladder. Chant Chui, *chuwee . . .* Feel the healing sound vibrate your Urinary Bladder. Repeat three times or more.

6. Become aware of your Kidney Family. Chant Chui, *chuwee . . .* Feel the healing sound vibrate your Ears, Kidneys, and Urinary Bladder. Repeat three times or more.

7. Continue to feel the vibration after the chanting ends.

8. Nourish your Ears, Kidneys, and Urinary Bladder. *I am in Qi; Qi is in me.*

Exercise 18: Awaken Your San Jiao Family

San Jiao Family

- Chant: Xi
- Healing sound: *Sheeee . . .*
- Mother: Pericardium
- Father: San Jiao
- Child: Face

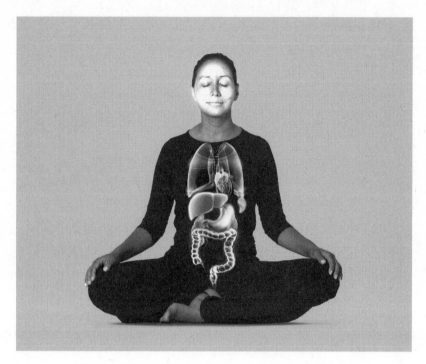

Figure 5.6: Fascia Covering Organs, Pericardium, and Face

Exercise Summary

The sixth and final healing sound in the series is the San Jiao Family Chant Xi, pronounced *she*. San Jiao, also called the Triple Warmer or the Triple Energizer, includes the fascia and interstitial fluids that cover the Organs. The fascia in the body cavity divides the Organs into three sections. The Upper Jiao includes the Heart and the Lungs, which relate to respiration and circulation. The Middle Jiao connects the Organs of digestion, the stomach, and spleen. The Lower Jiao includes the Liver and Gallbladder, the Small Intestine, the Large Intestines as well as the Kidneys, and the Urinary Bladder.

The Pericardium is a two-layered sac filled with fluid that acts as a barrier around the Heart and protects it both physically and chemically.

The Face is the child of San Jiao. The Face includes the Eyes, Tongue, Mouth and Lips, Nose, and Ears. The Pericardium is the mother of the Face and San Jiao is the father of the Face.

The San Jiao healing sound is *sheeee* . . . As you chant *sheeee* . . . feel your entire Face vibrate. Then direct Xi to the esophagus in the back of your throat, and from there, down the body cavity. Vibrate the Lungs, the Heart, the Stomach and Spleen, the Liver and Gallbladder, the Small Intestine and the Large Intestine all the way to the anus. Feel your entire body cavity vibrating down to the pelvic floor as you chant Xi. Direct Xi to the Pericardium, *sheeee* . . . Feel the entire San Jiao Family vibrate as you chant Xi. Continue to feel the vibration after the chanting ends.

Exercise Instruction

The formal instructions for this exercise are detailed below.

1. Adopt Natural Sitting Posture and close your eyes gently.

2. Practice Taiji Breathing for three cycles until your mind is calm.

3. Become aware of your Face. Chant Si, *sheeee* . . . Feel the healing sound vibrate your Face. Repeat three times or more.

4. Become aware of your San Jiao. Chant Si, *sheeee* . . . Feel the healing sound vibrate your San Jiao. Repeat three times or more.

5. Become aware of your Pericardium. Chant Si, *sheeee* . . . Feel the healing sound vibrate your Pericardium. Repeat three times or more.

6. Become aware of your San Jiao Family. Chant Si, *sheeee* . . . Feel the healing sound vibrate your Face, San Jiao, and Pericardium. Repeat three times or more.

7. Continue to feel the vibration after the chanting ends.

8. Nourish your Face, San Jiao, and Pericardium. *I am in Qi; Qi is in me.*

The table below summarizes the new associations we have established with the Six Organ Families.

Organ Family	Child	Mother	Father	Chant	Healing Sound
Liver	Eyes	Liver	Gallbladder	Xu	*Shewww . . .*
Heart	Tongue	Heart	Small Intestine	Ha	*Haaaaa . . .*
Spleen	Mouth and Lips	Spleen	Stomach	Hu	*Whoooo . . .*
Lung	Nose	Lungs	Large Intestine	Si	*Szzzzz . . .*
Kidney	Ears	Kidneys	Urinary Bladder	Chui	*Chuwee . . .*
San Jiao	Face	Pericardium	San Jiao	Xi	*Sheeee . . .*

Exercise 19: Awaken the Six Organ Families

This exercise combines the previous six exercises and awakens all Six Organ Families in one sitting. After chanting, you may feel waves of heat or cold, heaviness or lightness, and the feeling of crawling ants moving through some parts of your body. These are the sensations of Qi energy awakening an Organ or possibly releasing trapped energy. Should any unusual sensations arise, allow them to pass. If any emotions arise, let them pass. If any experience you encounter becomes overwhelming, simply open your eyes and breathe naturally. Go for a walk. After some time, the blockages will diminish, and these sensations will decrease.

1. Adopt Natural Sitting Posture and close your eyes gently.

2. Practice Taiji Breathing for three cycles until your mind is calm.

3. Become aware of your Liver Family. Chant Xu, *shewww* . . .
   Feel the healing sound vibrate your Eyes, Liver, and
   Gallbladder. Repeat three times or more.

4. Become aware of your Heart Family. Chant Ha, *haaaaa* . . .
   Feel the healing sound vibrate your Tongue, Heart, and
   Small Intestine. Repeat three times or more.

5. Become aware of your Spleen Family. Chant Hu, *whoooo* . . .
   Feel the healing sound vibrate your Mouth and Lips, Spleen,
   and Stomach. Repeat three times or more.

6. Become aware of your Lung Family. Chant Si, *szzzzz* . . .
   Feel the healing sound vibrate your Nose, Lungs, and Large
   Intestine. Repeat three times or more.

7. Become aware of your Kidney Family. Chant Chui,
   chuwee . . . Feel the healing sound vibrate your Ears, Kidneys,
   and Urinary Bladder. Repeat three times or more.

8. Become aware of your San Jiao Family. Chant Si, *sheeee* . . .
   Feel the healing sound vibrate your Face, San Jiao, and
   Pericardium. Repeat three times or more.

9. Continue to feel the vibration after the chanting ends.
   Feel all the Organ Families vibrating. Relax and enjoy the
   experience.

10. Nourish your Qi. *I am in Qi; Qi is in me.*

Healing and Empowering the Organs

Awakening the Six Organ Families concludes the first of three parts
that make up The Six Healing Sounds Meditation. Once you become
proficient at awakening an Organ and experience it buzzing with Qi
energy, you are ready to begin the next parts of the practice, *Healing the*

Organs and *Empowering the Organs.* While Awakening the Organs can be practiced on its own, Healing and Empowering the Organs should be practiced together. These two parts of the practice work as a unit and are presented together.

We begin by exploring the technique we use for Healing the Organs. To Heal an Organ, we "enter" the Organ, scan the organ, and heal it from within by *whispering* its healing sound. What does it mean to "enter" the Organ? Qi energy is the force that mediates between experiencing ourselves as an object and a subject. Earlier, you tapped your Liver and felt it objectively. Just like you can tap your knee or your chin. Any part of the body can be experienced objectively. But once we awaken a part of the body by infusing it with Qi energy, we are able to experience it subjectively. We can enter that part of the body with our mind.

A simple experiment clarifies this idea. Touch your right hand with your left hand as you would touch any object. Feel the contour of the bones, the texture of the skin and nails. Now rub your hands together until your hand is buzzing with Qi. Close your eyes and experience your right hand as a subject. Allow your awareness to penetrate deeply into your hand. Become aware of the inside of your hand.

A well-known principle of Daoist meditation is that *mind follows Qi.* Once a part of your body is buzzing with energy, your mind can penetrate it. That is how an object becomes a subject. This principle applies to energy healing in general. When an energy healer's hands are full of Qi, they become like sonar waves that are used to probe the depth of the ocean. A healer places her physical hands on the body of a patient, and she is able to probe the inside of the body with her energy hands. She can scan the energy field and find obstructions, then heal the patient by removing the obstructions that are impeding proper Qi flow.

Similarly, once we activate an Organ by chanting the healing sound, we can penetrate the Organ with our mind, scan for blockages, and heal the Organ by restoring healthy Qi flow. If we chant Si and energize our Lungs, for example, our mind can penetrate our Lungs, scan them for repressed emotions and other obstructions, and heal the Lungs by releasing the negativity trapped inside.

Once you activate the Lungs through chanting Xi and you feel your Lung Qi buzzing, simply allow your mind to travel inside your Lungs and become aware of any negative sensations. You might feel an area inside your Lungs that is dense or perceive spots that are dark or feel uncomfortable. You might experience trapped memories of sadness, old grievances, or the feeling of injustice arising in awareness. Any negative emotion associated with the Lungs can be stirred as your mind probes the Lungs. It is essential not to repress any negative feeling that arises. This is not the time for judging, analyzing, or evaluating. Love yourself and show compassion. Healing embraces negativity to release it. Pushing trapped energies further inside the Organ undermines the healing process.

The way that we release negative energy and heal an Organ is by whispering the healing sound of the Organ. In the case of the Lungs, we whisper Xi, *szzzzz* . . . Whispering has a cleansing effect. Whispering loosens, soothes, and facilitates release. As we whisper the healing sound, we are communicating to the Organ, "Let go of any energy that does not serve your highest good." "Release the past." "Everything will be alright." Whisper the healing sound gently. Whisper lovingly. Whisper and release the negativity. Surrender the negativity. Feel its grip slip. Stuck negative emotions consume energy. The part of you that is holding on to repressed emotions is exhausted. Let go. Let go. Whisper the healing sound and release. Whisper the healing sound and heal the Organ.

Negative energies sometimes release quickly, and sometimes the release may take a long time. There may be multiple layers of negativity and the healing process can be compared to paring the leaves of an artichoke. We peel off leaf after leaf until we get to the core. As you whisper the healing sound you may release one instance of repressed energy, and then another presents itself for healing. And then another, and another, until all the trapped negativity is released. As we practice whispering, we are delving deeper into the Organ, stretching further back in time, healing older wounds, some of which are rooted in early childhood and may not make sense. Some wounds may even be karmic and rooted in past lives. Don't try to make sense of the energies or images that arise. When a negative memory or sensation arises, whisper it out of your system.

To practice Healing the Organs, you should not be under the influence of drugs or alcohol. Your mind must be clear and steady. Awareness must be sharp and relaxed. If you are under psychiatric care and taking drugs for a mental condition, please consult with your doctor before practicing because sometimes an emotional release can be intense. As negativity is released, the emotional energy that was trapped surges as it passes through you. If you are releasing anger, you may experience intense anger. If you are releasing fear, you may experience intense fear. Realize the difference between being angry and witnessing anger releasing. When a doctor lances a festering wound, a putrid smell fills the room. Releasing a festering emotional wound can also fill us with a putrid feeling. If a strong sensation arises as you release a negative emotion, allow the experience to pass. It will dissipate, and once it passes, you will feel lighter and more energized.

After we Heal an Organ by whispering, we Empower the Organ by *mouthing* the healing sound. If we ended the Six Healing Sounds with whispering, we might feel relieved of some negativity, but also depleted. So right after whispering, we repeat the healing sound again, but this time with an intention to empower the positive emotional quality of the organ, its Organ Virtue. The empowerment is accomplished by *mouthing* the healing sound. Move your mouth as though you were chanting or whispering, but don't make a sound. Whispering is done on the exhale and mouthing is done on the inhale. As you mouth the healing sound, perceive it subvocally.

Whereas chanting activates an Organ and gets it to vibrate, and whispering facilities the release of negative energy, mouthing draws in and absorbs. Whispering and mouthing represent opposite energetic dynamics. When we whisper and exhale, we push out, and when we mouth and inhale, we pull in. Let's imagine that you were praying for something negative to leave your life. It would be most effective to whisper the prayer. Let's imagine that you were praying for something positive to come into your life. It would be most effective to mouth the prayer. Try this experiment for yourself sometime. The difference between whispering and mouthing is remarkable.

Another way to visualize the difference between whispering and mouthing is as follows. When you whisper the healing sound, you are squeezing dirty water from a sponge. When you mouth the Organ Sound, the sponge is absorbing clean water. As you practice whispering, feel as though you are squeezing out the impurities and obstructions from the Organ. As you mouth, feel positive energy absorb into the Organ. Feel the Organ contract energetically when you whisper and expand energetically when you mouth.

As you mouth the healing sound, absorb the energy of the Universe into the Organ. As you mouth the healing sound, feel the Organ Virtue fill the Organ from within like fresh spring water. Feel the radiant energy of the Universe and the Organ Virtue empower the Organ. Feel the Organ radiating emotional well-being from within and without. After mouthing the Lung sound, for example, you should feel a field of radiant kindness permeating your Lungs that you can draw on throughout the day. Allow this kindness to motivate your actions and your words. As the Organ Virtues brighten your Higher Mind, you are filled with a sense of well-being that inspires goodwill.

In the section that follows, we detail the positive and negative qualities associated with each Organ Family. This information will help you navigate through the healing process and the empowerment of the Organs. Then we practice healing and empowering the Organ Families. We follow the same sequence previously established and begin with the Liver Family.

The Emotions of the Liver Family

The Voice of the Liver

The sequence begins with the Liver Family because the Liver Family is the Organ Pair that wants to be first the most. The Liver embodies the archetype of the General. Picture troops readying for a battle. They are scared. They are worried. Some of them will not survive. A foreboding sense of despair settles over them. The General gathers his soldiers and gives them a rousing speech. He fires them up with uplifting words. He inspires them and sparks enthusiasm. They roar with confidence.

They become convinced that they will emerge victorious. We cannot say how the battle will fare, but we can say that a good General will stack the odds on the side of victory by inspiring his troops with courage and valor. Another archetype associated with the Liver is the Coach who rouses the team at halftime, or the Professor who inspires her students with moving words. The voice that uplifts and inspires is the voice of the Liver. The voice that instills confidence and optimism is the voice of the Liver. If your Liver is healthy, you can reach into your reserve of Liver Qi and use that energy to inspire yourself and others.

When Liver Qi is dissonant, we tend to exaggerate and be unrealistic. We are overenthusiastic. We overpromise. And when we fail, we become frustrated. We shout and scream. We become overbearing, pompous, and self-righteous. We blame others. Our egos inflate and we become insufferable. A loud voice that is overreaching and heavy-handed is the voice of a repressed Liver.

The Voice of the Gallbladder

Previously, we explored the courageous nature of the Gallbladder, the Brave Warrior. In battle, second place is not an option. The ability to initiate bold action is imperative. The Gallbladder speaks in a strong voice. It is a daunting voice that is not afraid to push forward despite the risk. The Gallbladder dares and provokes. It challenges and competes. The ability to push yourself and others to go further faster is drawing on Gallbladder Qi.

When Gallbladder Qi is repressed, we are unable to summon courage or initiative. We become timid and cowardly. We act boldly in situations that don't require courage and become Aggressive Bullies. We become reckless in trivial ways, endangering others or ourselves for no good reason. Flirting with danger by driving too fast on a highway is an example of negative Gallbladder Qi. It doesn't take courage to mindlessly press on the gas pedal and endanger others. When we start to sound like a drill sergeant booming orders and instilling fear in others, our Gallbladder voice is communicating imbalance. Dissonant Gallbladder Qi creates stress, conflict, and strife that serves no good purpose.

The Voice of the Liver Family

As an Organ Pair, the Liver and Gallbladder transform into the Warrior General who speaks with strategic insight and undaunted courage. This combination is attracted to risk and engages it head-on. The voice of the Liver Family inspires and pushes us to stretch the horizon of possibility. This combination welcomes adventure and danger. It fires up the mind with thoughts of expansion and speaks rousing words that drive us to action and victory.

The table below summarizes the emotional qualities of the Liver Family.

Liver Family	Negative Emotion	Positive Emotion	Archetype
Liver	Frustration	Enthusiasm	General
Gallbladder	Anger	Courage	Warrior
Liver and Gallbladder	Self-righteous anger	Encouraging optimism	Warrior General

---

Exercise 20: Heal and Empower Your Liver Family

Part 1

1. Adopt Natural Sitting Posture and practice Taiji Breathing for three cycles or more until your mind is calm.

2. Awaken your Liver by chanting Xu. Repeat three times or more.

3. Become aware of your Liver vibrating with Qi. Feel your awareness penetrate your Liver. Feel the spaciousness of your Liver. Abide in that spaciousness.

4. Whisper *shewww* . . . Whisper the healing sound at least three times. Probe your Liver. If you encounter any negative

energy or sensation, whisper *shewww* . . . Whisper in a gentle and caring way. Release frustration or any other negative emotion that arises. Keep on whispering the healing sound at your own speed until you are ready to move on.

5. Become aware of your Liver vibrating with Qi. Mouth *shewww* . . . Feel your Liver filling with positive emotional energy. Feel the qualities of enthusiasm, optimism, and hope fill your Liver. As you continue to mouth *shewww* . . . feel the positive qualities of the Liver growing stronger. Keep on mouthing the healing sound at your own speed until you are ready to move on.

6. Inhale and empower your Liver by absorbing Universal Qi, and exhale. Repeat three times or more, then relax and abide in the bliss of your Liver for as long as desired.

Part 2

7. Awaken your Gallbladder by chanting Xu. Repeat three times or more.

8. Become aware of your Gallbladder vibrating with Qi. Feel your awareness penetrate your Gallbladder. Feel the spaciousness of your Gallbladder. Abide in that spaciousness.

9. Whisper *shewww* . . . Whisper the healing sound at least three times. Probe your Gallbladder. If you encounter any negative energy or sensation, whisper *shewww* . . . Whisper in a gentle and caring way. Release anger or any other negative emotion that arises. Keep on whispering the healing sound at your own speed until you are ready to move on.

10. Become aware of your Gallbladder vibrating with Qi. Mouth *shewww* . . . Feel your Gallbladder filling with positive emotional energy. Feel the qualities of courage, bravery, and audacity fill your Gallbladder. As you continue to mouth *shewww* . . . feel the positive qualities of the Gallbladder

growing stronger. Keep on mouthing the healing sound at your own speed until you are ready to move on.

11. Inhale and empower your Gallbladder by absorbing Universal Qi, and exhale. Repeat three times or more, then relax and abide in the bliss of your Gallbladder for as long as desired.

Part 3

12. Nourish your Liver, Gallbladder, and Eyes. *I am in Qi; Qi is in me.*

The Emotions of the Heart Family

The Voice of the Heart

The Heart is the mother of the Tongue and the voices of all the Organs pass through the Heart on the way to the Tongue. All aspects of our mind must clear our Heart on the way to the Tongue. We speak our mind through our Heart. The Heart colors all voices on their way to the Tongue, and for this reason, the Heart is the central hub of consciousness.

We speak through the Heart, but the Heart also has its own voice. The Heart is the Emperor of the Organs. The voice of the Emperor communicates honor and dignity. Imagine a movie star walking into a restaurant. She is in the spotlight and all eyes turn toward her. Her presence brightens the room. Faces smile. Attention hovers around her. She is the center of attention. You don't have to literally be an Emperor to feel like one. Imagine being stopped on the street and asked a random question by a television crew. Now you're the Emperor. The camera is focused on you. A microphone is aimed at your mouth. People are paying attention. When our Heart Qi is healthy and strong, we are able to hold the center of attention. We feel comfortable in the spotlight. Our complexion turns rosy red, and we smile and glow when we are admired. Our voice is upbeat, and we are full of good cheer. Laughter comes easy. When our Heart Qi is healthy and strong, the voice of the Heart projects radiance and light. If the sun could speak, it would sound like the Heart.

When Heart Qi is dissonant, the Emperor becomes the Tyrant who demands attention. A negative Heart can become torridly oppressive. The generosity of the Heart turns to cruelty and honor turns to arrogance. The voice of joy becomes the overbearing voice of domination. The voice of hatred is a voice spoken by a wounded Heart. A repressed Heart can also be weak and unimposing. Picture a voice that lacks confidence and can't hold the center of attention. A deficient Heart has thin skin and finds offense at the slightest provocation. A pallid face that can't muster a glorious smile when that camera crew is filming is the clearest indication of a repressed Heart.

The Voice of the Small Intestine

The Small Intestine is the Decision-Maker that separates nutrients from waste material as food is processed in the digestive tract. The ability to prioritize and distinguish between the wheat and the chaff is a quality associated with healthy Small Intestine Qi. The Small Intestine is the voice that decides between what is useful and what is useless. The Small Intestine says yes to one thing and no to another. It ranks, makes lists, and prioritizes. The voice of the Small Intestine communicates precision and efficiency. Decisions that require discernment are governed by the Small Intestine.

When Small Intestine Qi is dissonant, we make undiscriminating decisions that lead to messy outcomes. A repressed Small Intestine cannot distinguish the baby from the bathwater. The baby is treated like the dirty water. The dirty water is treated like the baby. Dissonant Small Intestine Qi is unable to discern what is valuable and what is not. Priorities are inverted. Unforced errors are made, and as a result, we second guess ourselves incessantly. We become self-doubters and skeptics. Unhealthy Small Intestine Qi shifts the blame by finding fault in others. The dissonant Small Intestine speaks in an annoying voice that criticizes endlessly. It nags. It blames. The repressed Small Intestine looks down on others contemptuously. It is the voice of discrimination and prejudice.

The Voice of the Heart Family

As an Organ Pair, the healthy Heart and Small Intestine give rise to a voice that commands attention and makes decisions. This is the voice of the Discerning Emperor. He has the final say and he speaks on behalf of the entire kingdom. This voice cuts through confusion and offers clarity. It is an honorable and insightful voice. The voice of the Heart Family speaks in a powerful voice that radiates competence and is judicious and impartial. People cheer a noble-minded leader who offers warmth and chases away the gray clouds of confusion. The voice of the Heart Family is the sensible voice of the Discerning Emperor who the people love and admire.

Heart Family	Negative Emotion	Positive Emotion	Archetype
Heart	Arrogance	Nobility	Emperor
Small Intestine	Faultfinding	Discernment	Decision-Maker
Heart and Small Intestine	Arrogant criticism	Noble choices	Discerning Emperor

Exercise 21: Heal and Empower Your Heart Family

Note: Please be very gentle, slow, and patient when meditating on your Heart.

Part 1

1. Adopt Natural Sitting Posture and practice Taiji Breathing for three cycles or more until your mind is calm.

2. Awaken your Heart by chanting Ha. Repeat three times or more.

3. Become aware of your Heart vibrating with Qi. Feel your awareness penetrate your Heart. Feel the spaciousness of your Heart. Abide in that spaciousness.

4. Whisper *haaaaa* . . . Whisper the healing sound at least three times. Probe your Heart. If you encounter any negative energy or sensation, whisper *haaaaa* . . . Whisper in a gentle and caring way. Release arrogance, hatred, or any other negative emotion that arises. Keep on whispering the healing sound at your own speed until you are ready to move on.

5. Become aware of your Heart vibrating with Qi. Mouth *haaaaa* . . . Feel your Heart filling with positive emotional energy. Feel the qualities of joy, nobility, and generosity fill your Heart. As you continue to mouth *haaaaa* . . . feel the positive qualities of the Heart growing stronger. Keep on mouthing the healing sound at your own speed until you are ready to move on.

6. Inhale and empower your Heart by absorbing Universal Qi, and exhale. Repeat three times or more, then relax and abide in the bliss of your Heart for as long as desired.

Part 2

7. Awaken your Small Intestine by chanting Ha. Repeat three times or more.

8. Become aware of your Small Intestine vibrating with Qi. Feel your awareness penetrate your Small Intestine. Feel the spaciousness of your Small Intestine. Abide in that spaciousness.

9. Whisper *haaaaa* . . . Whisper the healing sound at least three times. Probe your Small Intestine. If you encounter any negative energy or sensation, whisper *haaaaa* . . . Whisper in a gentle and caring way. Release self-doubt, prejudice, or any other negative emotion that arises. Keep on whispering the healing sound at your own speed until you are ready to move on.

10. Become aware of your Small Intestine vibrating with Qi. Mouth *haaaaa* . . . Feel your Small Intestine filling with positive emotional energy. Feel the qualities of discernment, precision, and efficiency fill your Small Intestine. As you continue to mouth *haaaaa* . . . feel the positive qualities of the Small Intestine growing stronger. Keep on mouthing the healing sound at your own speed until you are ready to move on.

11. Inhale and empower your Small Intestine by absorbing Universal Qi, and exhale. Repeat three times or more, then relax and abide in the bliss of your Small Intestine for as long as desired.

Part 3

12. Nourish your Heart, Small Intestine, and Tongue. *I am in Qi; Qi is in me.*

The Emotions of the Spleen Family

The Voice of the Spleen

The Spleen is the Communicator who ponders and wonders. Healthy Spleen Qi is expressed as the ability to move around and maneuver with the dynamism of a toddler. Mental movement and physical movement are both expressions of Spleen Qi. The tumbling gymnast and the nimble thinker, who delights in mental gymnastics, are both expressing the flexibility and dexterity of the Spleen. The Spleen speaks in a clear voice that questions certainty and is open to new possibilities. This voice explores options and is drawn by curiosity toward novelty and change. The Spleen is the aspect of the psyche that wants to learn and teach. It is the compelling voice that stretches the mind and broadens perspectives. When two people are engaged in a spellbinding conversation that stretches their minds, they are feeding each other Spleen Qi.

When Spleen Qi is dissonant, we become restless. We ruminate endlessly about trivial matters. We speak too much but say little of value. Our attention span is short, and we become distracted easily. We are more likely to stretch the facts and even make them up. A repressed Spleen spreads rumors and misinforms. It can cheat and con. It is an irresponsible and unreliable voice. The voice of the negative Spleen creates confusion or is itself confused. It is the tricky and fickle voice of the car salesman who can't be trusted.

The Voice of the Stomach

The Stomach is the Comforter. We seek comfort through the food that we eat. The animal sounds that you make when you are sitting in front of your favorite dish are made by the voice of your Stomach. Imagine using that same voice to communicate what stirs your appetite. Maybe you like sailboats, and when you see a nice sailboat, you speak of it in the appreciative tone of the Stomach. The Stomach appreciates quality and regulates taste. The Stomach speaks in the tones of contentment and pleasure. It responds to what we value. The voice of gratitude and satisfaction is the voice of the Stomach. When Stomach Qi is flowing, we feel secure and stable. We revel in the energy of abundance. A comforting voice emanates from the Stomach. This is the soothing voice that reassures everything will be all right.

When Stomach Qi is dissonant, we feel upset and dissatisfied. We lack a sense of reassurance. We feel as though we might go hungry tomorrow. The feeling of running out of money or resources unsettles Stomach Qi. When we feel as though we are standing on shaky ground, we tighten our grip on our possessions. We resist change. Repressed Stomach Qi can make us greedy. We become obsessed by the need for pleasure and accumulating material possessions. We lust for gratification but are never satisfied. We are hungry for more but can never get enough. A disgruntled voice is spoken by a repressed Stomach. Repressed Stomach Qi can also conflate laziness and comfort. After a heavy meal, we don't feel like doing anything. We become a couch potato. The voice of procrastination and slothfulness reflects a dissonant Stomach.

The Voice of the Spleen Family

As an Organ Pair, the healthy and integrated Stomach and Spleen give rise to the voice of the Reassuring Communicator. When we encounter a trustworthy voice that imparts valuable information, we are talking to someone with strong Spleen Family Qi. This is a reliable and insightful voice that instills a sense of comfort. When you enjoy speaking with someone who puts your mind at ease, that conversation is nourishing your Spleen Family Qi. When you are in the presence of a likable and supportive friend who offers a sense of reassurance, you are nurturing your Spleen Family Qi.

Spleen Family	Negative Emotion	Positive Emotion	Archetype
Spleen	Restlessness	Clarity	Communicator
Stomach	Dissatisfaction	Reliability	Comforter
Spleen and Stomach	Restless dissatisfaction	Pleasant conversation	Reassuring Communicator

Exercise 22: Heal and Empower Your Spleen Family

Part 1

1. Adopt Natural Sitting Posture and practice Taiji Breathing for three cycles or more until your mind is calm.

2. Awaken your Spleen by chanting Hu. Repeat three times or more.

3. Become aware of your Spleen vibrating with Qi. Feel your awareness penetrate your Spleen. Feel the spaciousness of your Spleen. Abide in that spaciousness.

4. Whisper *huuuuu* . . . Whisper the healing sound at least three times. Probe your Spleen. If you encounter any negative energy or sensation, whisper *huuuuu* . . . Whisper in a gentle and caring way. Release restlessness or any other negative emotion that arises. Keep on whispering the healing sound at your own speed until you are ready to move on.

5. Become aware of your Spleen vibrating with Qi. Mouth *huuuuu* . . . Feel your Spleen filling with positive emotional energy. Feel the qualities of clarity, adaptability, and dexterity fill your Spleen. As you continue to mouth *huuuuu* . . . feel the positive qualities of the Spleen growing stronger. Keep on mouthing the healing sound at your own speed until you are ready to move on.

6. Inhale and empower your Spleen by absorbing Universal Qi, and exhale. Repeat three times or more, then relax and abide in the bliss of your Spleen for as long as desired.

Part 2

7. Awaken your Stomach by chanting Hu. Repeat three times or more.

8. Become aware of your Stomach vibrating with Qi. Feel your awareness penetrate your Stomach. Feel the spaciousness of your Stomach. Abide in that spaciousness.

9. Whisper *huuuuu* . . . Whisper the healing sound at least three times. Probe your Stomach. If you encounter any negative energy or sensation, whisper *huuuuu* . . . Whisper in a gentle and caring way. Release dissatisfaction, lethargy, or any other negative emotion that arises. Keep on whispering the healing sound at your own speed until you are ready to move on.

10. Become aware of your Stomach vibrating with Qi. Mouth *huuuuu* . . . Feel your Stomach filling with positive emotional energy. Feel the qualities of satisfaction, comfort, and stability fill your Stomach. As you continue to mouth *huuuuu* . . . feel the positive qualities of the Stomach growing stronger. Keep on mouthing the healing sound at your own speed until you are ready to move on.

11. Inhale and empower your Stomach by absorbing Universal Qi, and exhale. Repeat three times or more, then relax and abide in the bliss of your Stomach for as long as desired.

Part 3

12. Nourish your Spleen, Stomach, and Tongue. *I am in Qi; Qi is in me.*

The Emotions of the Lung Family

The Voice of the Lungs

The Lungs are the Peacemakers who speak in a considerate and measured tone. The Lungs are delicate Organs that react with nuance and subtlety. They are kind and sympathetic. The voice of the Lungs is an agreeable voice that you can trust. It is an accommodating voice. It is a friendly voice. The voice of the Lungs is inviting. The host who greets you in a welcoming tone and is attentive to your needs is communicating in the voice of the Lungs. The Lungs also hold our grief, and vibrant Lung Qi enables us to release our sadness through tears and a sigh. After we cry and sigh, we let go of the tension that we are holding. We can breathe properly again and replenish our Lungs on the next inhale.

When Lung Qi is repressed, our Lungs are unable to release sadness. We can't sigh properly or reenergize our Lungs. Our chest cavity sags. We slump. We become the Morose Downer who is constantly depressed and fills the room with melancholy. This voice is tinged with sorrow.

With repressed Lung Qi, we bounce back like a deflated basketball. We lack pep. We fall into a pit of gloom and self-pity. Repressed Lung Qi can also become overly accommodating to garner sympathy and kindness. Repressed Lung Qi gives rise to the archetypes of the Appeaser and the Sycophant, who yearn for approval and kindness from others. But repressed kindness usually draws in abusive people who take advantage of weak boundaries and an overly agreeable personality. Repressed Lung Qi is perpetually filled with sadness and grievance.

The Voice of the Large Intestine

The Large Intestine purges waste material from the body. That toxic material ends up in the toilet and is flushed down as soon as it passes. We do not touch it. It smells bad. We avoid it. There are some charged emotional topics that we want to avoid like our waste. These taboo subjects make us feel uncomfortable. If we have betrayed someone or engaged in some shameful or illegal activity, we would prefer to keep our actions hidden. The Large Intestine is the voice that emanates from the bowels of the psyche and confronts that discomfort. It is the voice that draws us to the source of our discomfort so that we can let go of our dark past and heal. A good psychotherapist leads us to those shadowy emotional places where we hold emotional waste and helps us to release those toxic energies. The voice of the Large Intestine purges those places within us that are rotting and helps heal our festering wounds.

Toxicity exists within us and it also exists in society. The whistleblower that exposes institutional corruption is harnessing Large Intestine Qi when revealing the ugly truth. Any truthteller that shines light on shameful abuse is speaking in the voice of the Large Intestine. Healthy Large intestine Qi is like the tank lever we press to flush the toilet. The feeling of relief that we experience after a healthy bowel movement and the feeling of relief that we experience after releasing toxic emotional waste are similar. After the Large Intestine flushes the emotional waste material, we feel purged, light, and transformed.

When Large Intestine Qi is not flowing smoothly, emotional waste material is not being processed properly and we communicate emotional diarrhea or constipation. The voice of diarrhea is the voice that blurts out toxic words intended to hurt. Hurtful words often have a kernel of truth but become destructive when they are communicated with ill will. A disturbed Large Intestine can give rise to the archetype of the Monster. Repressed Large Intestine Qi can also backflow and flood the mind with disgusting dark thoughts. The constipated voice is a voice that holds back the truth in order to avoid discomfort. This constriction of Large Intestine Qi torments the soul as rage ferments in the bowels of the psyche. When Large Intestine Qi is repressed, we feel as though we are drowning in a cesspool.

The Voice of the Lung Family

As an Organ Pair, the Lungs and the Large Intestine give rise to the archetype of the Trusted Soulmate. This Organ Pair generates a voice that communicates the hard truth diplomatically. When you hear this voice, you may not like what is being said, but you appreciate the honesty. Intensity and kindness both resonate when this voice speaks. This voice cuts like a knife to the bone. It exposes the festering core and sympathizes with the pain it exposes. This is a sympathetic voice with the power to change you. This voice takes you to the edge of your comfort zone and coaxes you to kindly take another step.

Lung Family	Negative Emotion	Positive Emotion	Archetype
Lungs	Sadness	Kindness	Diplomat
Large Intestine	Disgust	Honesty	Therapist
Lung and Large Intestine	Gloomy depression	Kind intensity	Trusted Soulmate

Exercise 23: Heal and Empower Your Lung Family

Part 1

1. Adopt Natural Sitting Posture and practice Taiji Breathing for three cycles or more until your mind is calm.

2. Awaken your Lungs by chanting Si. Repeat three times or more.

3. Become aware of your Lungs vibrating with Qi. Feel your awareness penetrate your Lungs. Feel the spaciousness of your Lungs. Abide in that spaciousness.

4. Whisper *szzzzz* . . . Whisper the healing sound at least three times. Probe your Lungs. If you encounter any negative energy or sensation, whisper *szzzzz* . . . Whisper in a gentle and caring way. Release sadness or any other negative emotion that arises. Keep on whispering the healing sound at your own speed until you are ready to move on.

5. Become aware of your Lungs vibrating with Qi. Mouth *szzzzz* . . . Feel your Lungs filling with positive emotional energy. Feel the qualities of kindness, consideration, and sympathy fill your Lungs. As you continue to mouth *szzzzz* . . . feel the positive qualities of the Lungs growing stronger. Keep on mouthing the healing sound at your own speed until you are ready to move on.

6. Inhale and empower your Lungs by absorbing Universal Qi, and exhale. Repeat three times or more, then relax and abide in the bliss of your Lungs for as long as desired.

Part 2

7. Awaken your Large Intestine by chanting Si. Repeat three times or more.

8. Become aware of your Large Intestine vibrating with Qi. Feel your awareness penetrate your Large Intestine. Feel the spaciousness of your Large Intestine. Abide in that spaciousness.

9. Whisper *szzzzz* . . . Whisper the healing sound at least three times. Probe your Large Intestine. If you encounter any negative energy or sensation, whisper *szzzzz* . . . Whisper in a gentle and caring way. Release disgust, betrayal, or any other negative emotion that arises. Keep on whispering the healing sound at your own speed until you are ready to move on.

10. Become aware of your Large Intestine vibrating with Qi. Mouth *szzzzz* . . . Feel your Large Intestine filling with positive emotional energy. Feel the qualities of honesty, intensity, and purgation fill your Large Intestine. As you continue to mouth *szzzzz* . . . feel the positive qualities of the Large Intestine growing stronger. Keep on mouthing the healing sound at your own speed until you are ready to move on.

11. Inhale and empower your Large Intestine by absorbing Universal Qi, and exhale. Repeat three times or more, then relax and abide in the bliss of your Large Intestine for as long as desired.

Part 3

12. Nourish your Lungs, Large Intestine, and Nose. *I am in Qi; Qi is in me.*

The Emotions of the Kidney Family

The Voice of the Kidneys

The Kidneys embody the voice of the Wise Elder. That voice is cautious and calculated. It is measured and reserved. The voice of the Kidneys is a serious voice that commands respect. It is a responsible voice that delivers instructions and executes orders. When you are speaking to an authority figure, like a doctor or a customs official at the airport, you are communicating Kidney energy. Kidney Qi has the capacity to persevere. When you face a monumental task, it is Kidney Qi that is invoked. Your ambition and tenacity to reach the summit of excellence is an expression of your Kidneys. The voice of steely determination that does not waver in the face of hardship belongs to the Kidneys. When Kidney Qi is strong, success in a long-term endeavor is more likely.

When Kidney Qi is deficient, we feel fatigued. Our voice diminishes. We are ineffective and tire easily. Our stamina is low, and we groan when we need to summon a burst of energy to get a demanding task accomplished. Kidneys become weary from overwork and constant pressure. Carrying a burden for a long time without recuperative rest weakens the Kidneys. When the Kidneys are imbalanced, the voice we project carries a negative tone. The pessimistic voice of failure belongs to the repressed Kidneys.

The Voice of the Urinary Bladder

Pressure builds up in the Urinary Bladder as the toxins produced by the Kidneys fill it with urine. At some point, we feel the urge to urinate, and when we do, we feel relieved. The relief we experience from too much pressure captures the positive feeling associated with the Urinary Bladder. When we find ourselves in situations that force us to conform against our will, we activate Urinary Bladder Qi. We become "pissed off" and speak in a defiant voice that opposes limitation and seeks relief from oppression. The voice of the Urinary Bladder is the voice of the activist who seeks relief from oppressive societal rules. It is also the voice of the Innovator who offers a vision of a better future free of the limitations of the present. When we lead inauthentic lives, crushing pressure builds internally and we seek relief by expressing our authentic self. The voice of authenticity is the voice of the Urinary Bladder. This voice is forward-thinking and thrives on progress. It can be oppositional and confrontational. It focuses on a better tomorrow. The voice of the Urinary Bladder is the voice of freedom.

When the Urinary Bladder is bursting with pressure, we feel on edge. Imagine not being able to relieve your bladder, ever. Imagine living under that oppression day after day with no end in sight. Emotionally, you would also be bursting at the seams. The voice of a repressed Urinary bladder is inauthentic and fearful. It conforms to authority but builds resentment. It is a jealous voice that envies the freedom of others. It holds grudges against those who oppress. This voice can become erratic and rebellious. Or it can crumble into madness under a toxic load too heavy to bear. A dissonant Urinary Bladder speaks in the broken voice of a repressed human leading an inauthentic life. An impostor whose voice lacks authenticity and gives up too easily in the face of hardship is speaking through a weak Urinary Bladder.

The Voice of the Kidney Family

As an Organ Pair, the Kidneys and the Urinary Bladder give rise to the archetype of the Tough Old Bird. This combination speaks in a resilient voice that never gives up. It is an ambitious voice that expresses itself freely. It becomes its own authority. The voice of the Kidneys is dignified and willful. It is a steely voice that cannot be bent by outside pressure. It is fearless and committed. It is disciplined and determined. This voice is willing to step outside the box to find a better box. It is an authentic voice that is respected even by those who oppose what it has to say.

Kidney Family	Negative Emotion	Positive Emotion	Archetype
Kidneys	Fear	Caution	Elder
Urinary Bladder	Resentment	Authenticity	Innovator
Kidneys and Urinary Bladder	Fear and oppression	Respect and resilience	Tough Old Bird

Exercise 24: Heal and Empower Your Kidney Family

Part 1

1. Adopt Natural Sitting Posture and practice Taiji Breathing for three cycles or more until your mind is calm.

2. Awaken your Kidneys by chanting Chui. Repeat three times or more.

3. Become aware of your Kidneys vibrating with Qi. Feel your awareness penetrate your Lungs. Feel the spaciousness of your Kidneys. Abide in that spaciousness.

4. Whisper *chuwee* . . . Whisper the healing sound at least three times. Probe your Kidneys. If you encounter any negative energy or sensation, whisper *chuwee* . . . Whisper in a gentle and caring way. Release the feeling of failure or any other negative emotion that arises. Keep on whispering the healing sound at your own speed until you are ready to move on.

5. Become aware of your Kidneys vibrating with Qi. Mouth *chuwee* . . . Feel your Kidneys filling with positive emotional energy. Feel the qualities of resilience, caution, and discipline fill your Kidneys. As you continue to mouth *chuwee* . . . feel the positive qualities of the Kidneys growing stronger. Keep on mouthing the healing sound at your own speed until you are ready to move on.

6. Inhale and empower your Kidneys by absorbing Universal Qi, and exhale. Repeat three times or more, then relax and abide in the bliss of your Kidneys for as long as desired.

Part 2

7. Awaken your Urinary Bladder by chanting Chui. Repeat three times or more.

8. Become aware of your Urinary Bladder vibrating with Qi. Feel your awareness penetrate your Urinary Bladder. Feel the spaciousness of your Urinary Bladder. Abide in that spaciousness.

9. Whisper *chuwee* . . . Whisper the healing sound at least three times. Probe your Urinary Bladder. If you encounter any negative energy or sensation, whisper *chuwee* . . . Whisper in a gentle and caring way. Release resentment or any other negative emotion that arises. Keep on whispering the healing sound at your own speed until you are ready to move on.

10. Become aware of your Urinary Bladder vibrating with Qi. Mouth *chuwee* . . . Feel your Urinary Bladder filling with positive emotional energy. Feel the qualities of authenticity, freedom, and innovation fill your Urinary Bladder. As you continue to mouth *chuwee* . . . feel the positive qualities of the Urinary Bladder growing stronger. Keep on mouthing the healing sound at your own speed until you are ready to move on.

11. Inhale and empower your Urinary Bladder by absorbing Universal Qi and exhale. Repeat three times or more, then relax and abide in the bliss of your Urinary Bladder for as long as desired.

Part 3

12. Nourish your Kidneys, Urinary Bladder, and Ears. *I am in Qi; Qi is in me.*

The Emotions of the San Jiao Family

The Voice of San Jiao

San Jiao, the fascia that covers the Organs, is the Conductor of the emotional orchestra. San Jiao orchestrates and harmonizes the voices of all the Organs. If an instrument is out of tune in an orchestra, the Conductor is responsible for pointing it out. If one of the Organ voices is discordant, San Jiao will point it out. Maybe your Kidneys are fatigued, and you groan a lot, or your Small Intestine is out of tune, and you nag too much. Possibly both of these Organs are simultaneously imbalanced, and you become a tiresome and critical naysayer. San Jiao regulates the capacity to pick up on our own negative energy and helps us regain emotional coherence. It also enables us to pick up on the energy of other people. San Jiao is our awareness of the whole in relation to the parts. San Jiao is the voice of empathy that understands which parts are not integrated. Imagine a portrait in which all the features match except for the eyes. They are too big for the face. Maybe Liver Family Qi is unintegrated. San Jiao is the voice that will recognize that flaw and attempt to correct it. San Jiao is the harmonious voice that strives for unity and wholeness.

When San Jiao is dissonant, the voices of the Organs don't communicate properly. They lack coordination. Before an orchestra begins to produce consonant music, the musicians each tune their instrument and produce a cacophony of sounds. When San Jiao is imbalanced, our psyche becomes a cacophony of discordant voices that lack coherence. We fragment internally. We contradict ourselves. When we lack San Jiao awareness, we produce clunky music. People experience us as inconsistent and hypocritical. When we become incoherent and befuddling, San Jiao is very possibly the root of the problem. When we undermine our self-interest and sabotage ourselves consistently, we are expressing an unhealthy San Jiao pattern of behavior. Without healthy San Jiao Qi, we feel helpless and lost.

The Voice of the Pericardium

The Pericardium is the Heart protector. It plays the role of the loyal Bodyguard to the Emperor. The Pericardium can also be envisioned as a mother that protects her vulnerable child. The Heart is extremely sensitive and once it is harmed, the entire psyche and mind become disturbed. Protecting and nurturing the Heart are the imperative functions served by the Pericardium. The Pericardium is a caring voice that shields with the ferocity of a mama bear. It also censors the voices that reach the Heart. It has veto power over the voices of the other Organs. It can repress negative emotions or hold them in check. It is the container that holds the psyche together. The Pericardium holds our emotions together like a soup bowl that is too hot to drink. It lets us simmer down and keeps us from burning ourselves and others with inappropriate words and actions.

When the Pericardium is imbalanced, we lack the capacity to contain our emotions wisely. Words are spoken that we later regret. We "burn" our Tongue with inappropriate words or actions. When the Pericardium is dissonant, our "deflector shield" malfunctions and the Heart becomes vulnerable to the hurtful words of others. We cannot defend ourselves properly and we become overly defensive. We become manic and over-sensitive. In a panic, the Pericardium can shut down the psyche like a clam and keep the Heart safe but invisible. When we want to say something but are held back by shyness or inhibition, our voice is being held back by an overly protective Pericardium. The Pericardium has the power to repress other emotions. When our voice is inhibited or maniacal, the Pericardium is the root of the problem.

The Voice of the San Jiao Family

As an Organ Pair, San Jiao and the Pericardium bring the qualities of care, protection, and harmony to the psyche. Both Organs envelop, contain, and unify the psyche, awakening a deep sense of emotional wholeness. The San Jiao Family speaks in the voice of the Compassionate Mother, who provides for all her children's needs and makes sure that they are safe. The San Jiao Family harmonizes and coordinates communication between the parts of the whole. The internal dialogue between the various voices of the Organs is mediated by the San Jiao Family. The San Jiao Family is the gravitational center that keeps all the Organs in harmonious orbit around our psychological center, the Heart.

San Jiao Family	Negative Emotion	Positive Emotion	Archetype
San Jiao	Fragmentation	Harmony	Conductor
Pericardium	Oversensitivity	Care	Bodyguard
San Jiao and Pericardium	Fragmented mania	Harmonious nurturing	Compassionate Mother

Exercise 25: Heal and Empower Your San Jiao Family

Part 1

1. Adopt Natural Sitting Posture and practice Taiji Breathing for three cycles or more until your mind is calm.

2. Awaken your San Jiao by chanting Xi. Repeat three times or more.

3. Become aware of your San Jiao vibrating with Qi. Feel your awareness penetrate San Jiao. Feel the spaciousness of San Jiao. Abide in that spaciousness.

4. Whisper *sheeee* . . . Whisper the healing sound at least three times. Probe San Jiao. If you encounter any negative energy or sensation, whisper *sheeee* . . . Whisper in a gentle and caring way. Release incoherence or any other negative emotion that arises. Keep on whispering the healing sound at your own speed until you are ready to move on.

5. Become aware of San Jiao vibrating with Qi. Mouth *sheeee* . . . Feel San Jiao filling with positive emotional energy. Feel the qualities of wholeness, harmony, and consistency fill San Jiao. As you continue to mouth *sheeee* . . . feel the positive qualities of San Jiao growing stronger. Keep on mouthing the healing sound at your own speed until you are ready to move on.

6. Inhale and empower San Jiao by absorbing Universal Qi, and exhale. Repeat three times or more, then relax and abide in the bliss of San Jiao for as long as desired.

Part 2

7. Awaken your Pericardium by chanting Xi. Repeat three times or more.

8. Become aware of your Pericardium vibrating with Qi. Feel your awareness penetrate your Pericardium. Feel the spaciousness of your Pericardium. Abide in that spaciousness.

9. Whisper *sheeee* . . . Whisper the healing sound at least three times. Probe your Pericardium. If you encounter any negative energy or sensation, whisper *sheeee* . . . Whisper in a gentle and caring way. Release inhibition, mania, or any other negative emotion that arises. Keep on whispering the healing sound at your own speed until you are ready to move on.

10. Become aware of your Pericardium vibrating with Qi. Mouth *sheeee* . . . Feel your Pericardium filling with positive emotional energy. Feel the qualities of care, loyalty, and protection fill your Pericardium. As you continue to mouth *sheeee* . . . feel the positive qualities of the Pericardium growing stronger. Keep on mouthing the healing sound at your own speed until you are ready to move on.

11. Inhale and empower your Pericardium by absorbing Universal Qi, and exhale. Repeat three times or more, then relax and abide in the bliss of your Pericardium for as long as desired.

Part 3

12. Nourish your San Jiao, Pericardium, and Face. *I am in Qi; Qi is in me.*

Exercise 26: The Six Healing Sounds Meditation

The Six Healings Sounds Meditation combines the awakening, healing, and mouthing of the Six Organ Families in one sitting. It combines all the exercises described in this chapter into one meditation. This meditation is a form of Daoist psychotherapy. As you practice the healing sounds and integrate your organ Qi, your psychological reality undergoes a transformation. Your emotional mind becomes integrated, and you are able to generate more goodwill.

Like all skills, mastering The Six Healing Sound Meditation takes time and practice. Some Organs may be more challenging to heal and empower than others. Some Organs may feel more constricted and require more practice. Sometimes you may chant a healing sound and drift into sleep. That's perfectly normal. Don't fight the urge to doze off. If you fall asleep while meditating, deep healings can take place. Sometimes, strong emotions may surge. As you release trapped Qi and old emotions, observe them impartially. If negative thoughts enter your mind as you practice, let them pass. Do not suppress those energies and force them back into your Organs. The negativity will dissipate and the next time you practice, there will be less of it.

As your practice develops, the Organ Virtues will become more palpable. They will fill your Organs with positive energy that will overflow into your interactions. Positive words will flow more freely, and positive actions will become easier for you to enact. Goodwill will arise even in the context of polarizing situations that might have triggered you previously. You will become increasingly sensitive to negative people. You will sense their negativity even if they are merely thinking a negative thought. As you progress, your mind will undergo a transformation and you will have a hard time generating negative thoughts. Your mind may stray from time to time, but you will feel uncomfortable in that space and quickly shift tracks.

Originally, Xiao Yao taught me The Six Healing Sound Meditation as a singular practice, but over time, I realized that breaking the practice into its component parts and mastering each part individually actually reduces the amount of time it takes for a student to master the practice. There are many nuances to this practice that can be glossed over when it is taught as a single practice in isolation. Once you have become familiar with the exercises in this chapter you may practice them in one continuous sitting.

The Six Healing Sounds Meditation begins with the San Jiao Family healing sound to activate the entire psyche and invite the archetype of the Compassionate Mother to guide and protect us as we heal and empower the Organs. The energy that we invite can assume the form of Guan Yin, Mother Mary, or any other caring motherly deity that represents the quality of divine protection. San Jiao energy is the safety net that we invoke at the start of the practice to create safe meditation space.

Part 1: Opening

1. Adopt Natural Sitting Posture and practice Taiji Breathing for three cycles or more until your mind is calm.

2. Awaken, heal, and empower the San Jiao Family by chanting, whispering, and mouthing the healing sound *sheeee* . . . Feel the qualities of safety, care, and compassion permeate the space within you and around you. Repeat three times or more.

Part 2: The Six Healing Sounds

3. Awaken, heal, and empower the Liver Family by chanting, whispering, and mouthing the healing sound *shewww* . . . Feel the qualities of courage and enthusiasm permeate the space within you and around you. Repeat three times or more.

4. Awaken, heal, and empower the Heart Family by chanting, whispering, and mouthing the healing sound *haaaaa* . . . Feel the qualities of confidence and discernment permeate the space within you and around you. Repeat three times or more.

5. Awaken, heal, and empower the Lung Family by chanting, whispering, and mouthing the healing sound *szzzzz* . . . Feel the qualities of kindness and relief permeate the space within you and around you. Repeat three times or more.

6. Awaken, heal, and empower the Kidney Family by chanting, whispering, and mouthing the healing sound *chuwee* . . . Feel the qualities of fear and resentment permeate the space within you and around you. Repeat three times or more.

7. Awaken, heal, and empower the San Jiao Family by chanting, whispering, and mouthing the healing sound *sheeee* . . . Feel the qualities of safety, care, and compassion permeate the space within you and around you. Repeat three times or more.

Closing

8. Nourish your Qi. *I am in Qi; Qi is in me.*

Once your Organs are awakened, healed, and empowered, your mind will overflow with the Organ Virtues. These qualities will ripple out into the world and harmonize your psyche and your relationships. Your Heart, the center of Higher Mind, will be filled with goodwill and appreciation, despite the adversity that you encounter day-to-day. Your Tongue will speak powerful words rooted in higher principles that will garner respect from others, even those who consider you an opponent. When your virtue consistently elicits admiration on the part of your enemies, it is a sign that you embody the nobility of Higher Mind and that you are ready to move on to the cultivation of Pure Mind, which follows next.

6

The Twelve Meridian Empowerment

The Pearl

Daoist mystical symbology and art hint at the mysterious imagery of a Pearl that is somehow related to meditation practice. The sages were not alluding to bright, lustrous, dense, and precious gems formed in the shell of an oyster that can be strung together to form a necklace. But ever practical, Daoist sages chose the imagery of a Pearl to allude the qualities of an *energy Pearl*, which is a bright, lustrous, dense, and precious energy presence made of concentrated Qi.

An energy Pearl is a concentrated point of Qi energy that we form with our mind and control through our intention. We form Pearls throughout the day without being aware of them. Have you ever heard a jingle that gets stuck in your mind? It repeats again and again in your mind, and if you are distracted for a few minutes it disappears but then returns again. Every time you make a mental note for later recall, you are also forming a Pearl. Anytime you concentrate mental or emotional energy, you are forming a Pearl.

We can leverage this natural process in the service of our meditation practice. Throughout the body we have a series of Energy Points that are energy rich. Imagine that I handed you a pair of magical goggles that allowed you to perceive the Energy Points spread throughout the body. You would see the human body light up like the lights of a city as seen from an airplane that is landing at night. You would notice that certain points are brighter than others. The point at the center of your palms, for example, would appear bright. The point at the top of your head would be luminous. The points at the ends of your finger and toe tips would be especially bright. Points by the wrist, elbows, shoulder, ankles, knees, and hips would also glow brightly. There would be many other points but most of those would shine less brightly. Daoist sages reasoned that forming a Pearl where the Energy Points shine brightest requires less effort and results in a Pearl that is more potent.

Another pattern that you would notice through the magic goggles is that these Energy Points are not scattered randomly. The points are connected by energy lines called Meridians that either begin or end at one of the Organs and extend to an extremity such as the fingertips or the toes. Visualize the Organ as a central railroad station, the Meridians as rail lines, and the Energy Points as stations along the way. Half the Meridians circulate Qi from an Organ to an extremity, and the other half circulate Qi from an extremity to an Organ. You would notice that there are twelve Meridians in each side of the body for a total of twenty-four Meridians. Even though the inside of the body is not symmetrical, the Meridian lines and their Energy Points are symmetrical. The Heart Meridian, for example, is the same on the left and right sides of the body despite the fact that we have one Heart and it is located on the left side of the body.

Meridians function like nerves or blood vessels that circulate blood and electric signals throughout the body, but Meridians circulate Qi rather than a physical substance. The concept of a Meridian sounds abstract and esoteric at first. Some may wonder why modern science has yet to uncover the Meridian network. After all, an anatomy student can cut open a body and identify blood vessels and nerves, but where are the Meridians? Until recently, the standard notion was that the Meridian system lacked a physical correlation. But a new theory is emerging that grounds ancient wisdom in modern science. As it turns out, the fascial sheets that extend throughout the body conduct a form of electricity called piezoelectricity. Furthermore, fascia possesses an organizational structure made up of swirls of connective tissue that correlate to a high degree with the location of the Energy Points described in acupuncture. Activating these points through pressure or needling has been shown to stimulate the circulation of piezoelectricity.

Some researchers speculate that the Meridians correlate to the major channels that circulate piezoelectricity within the fascial network, that Qi correlates to piezoelectricity, and that Energy Points correlate to the swirls within the fascial network. In the coming years, we can expect this fascinating theory to develop, and perhaps someday a scientific basis for acupuncture and Daoist meditation can be established.

Whichever way we choose to ground our understanding of the Meridians, Qi, and Energy Points, they can be experienced directly with relative ease, so you don't have to take anyone's word about their actuality. In a few paragraphs, you will awaken the Energy Point at the center of your palm, concentrate that Qi into a Pearl, and circulate that Pearl along an energy pathway to the end of your middle finger. Once you experience the dense and lingering presence of the Pearl circulating back and forth, you will realize that Pearls, Meridians, and Qi flow do not require an act of faith.

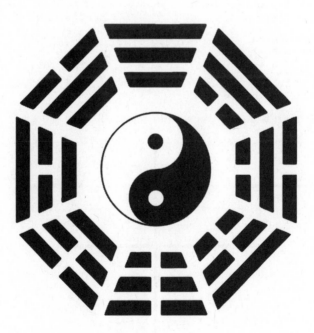

Figure 6.1: Bagua

The image of a Pearl can be transposed into another popular Daoist symbol that combines the Taiji with an octagonal figure known as a Bagua. The combination of these two symbols describes the formula for the formation of a Pearl. *Bagua plus Taiji equals a Pearl.* How do we interpret the meaning of this formula in a meaningful way?

Abstractly, a Bagua is an octagon—an eight-sided polygon such as the shape depicted below.

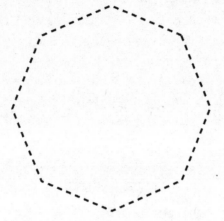

Figure 6.2: Octagon

To create a Bagua, we draw a plus sign . . .

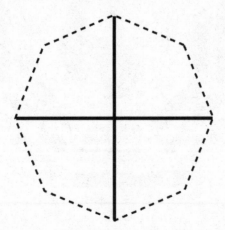

Figure 6.3: Octagon with Plus Sign

And a multiplication sign . . .

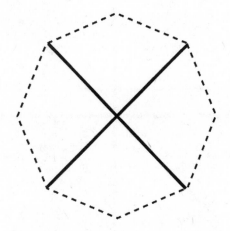

Figure 6.4: Octagon with Plus Multiplication Sign

And combine the two.

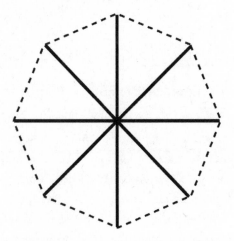

Figure 6.5: Octagon with Eight-Pointed Star

Technically, a Bagua is a plus sign combined with a multiplication sign. If we eliminate the dotted line, we end up with an eight-pointed star. The Bagua is implied by the eight-pointed star.

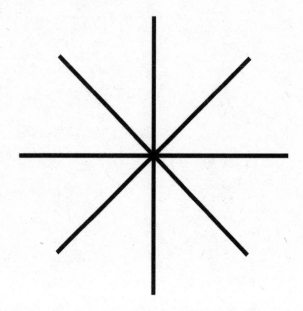

Figure 6.6: Eight-Pointed Star

Exercise 27: Form a Pearl

We are going to form this figure energetically at the center of your right hand to activate the Qi of the Energy Point at the center of your palm. Use your awareness to trace a plus sign. Trace the vertical line several times. You can use your eye movement to help direct the lines. As you move your eyes subtly up and down, feel the line form energetically on your palm. Then trace the horizontal line. Next, trace the two diagonal lines that make up the multiplication sign. Bring your awareness to the point where the lines intersect at the center. With a little practice, you will feel the center of your palm pulsating with energy. Repeat this process until you can discern the presence of Qi energy radiating from the star. Your palm may feel heavy, or it may pulsate energetically. Then move on to the next step.

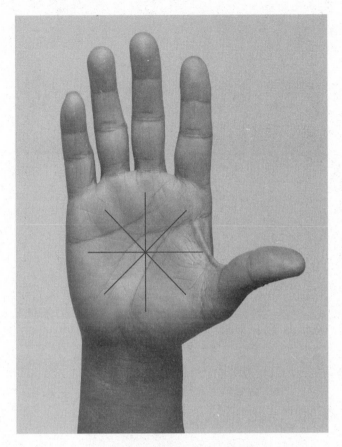

Figure 6.7: Eight-Pointed Star in Palm

Next, we are going to generate a Taiji in the form of a spiral that extends from the periphery of the Bagua toward the Energy Point at the center of your palm. A centripetal spiral is used to concentrate the Qi. The spiral can be clockwise or counterclockwise, whichever feels more natural. Use your eye movement to trace a circle around the Bagua and then spiral the Qi energy hovering over the star toward the center of your palm. Concentrate the Qi into a Pearl as it zeroes in on the Energy Point.

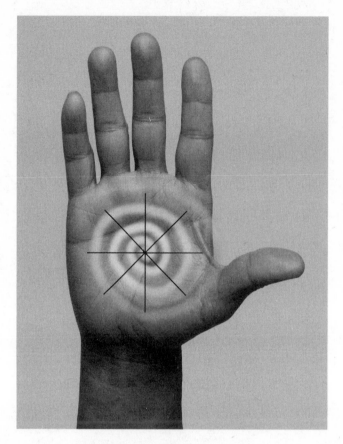

Figure 6.8: Palm with Star and Spiral

When the Taiji spiral reaches the center of your palm, you will feel a dense energetic presence that lingers in your palm even after you relax your awareness. Stop spiraling the Qi and become aware of the center of your palm. Do you feel a concentration of dense energy? Congratulations, you just formed a Pearl.

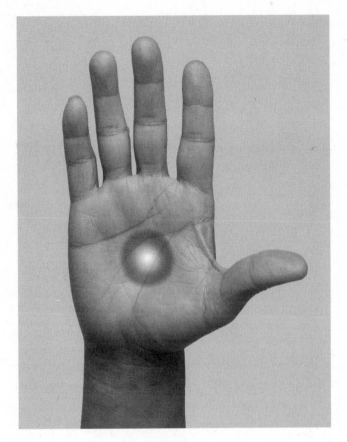

Figure 6.9: Pearl in Palm

The sensation of a Pearl should remain palpable even if your mind wanders for a short while. If you are distracted for a few moments and your attention returns to the Pearl, it should still be there. A Pearl is a dense and stable concentration of Qi. Compare your left hand to your right hand. Notice the difference between the two palms.

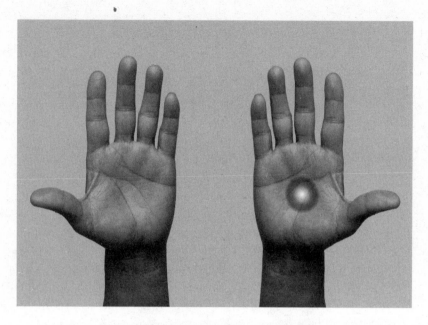

Figure 6.10: Comparing Left Palm to Right Palm

Next, use your awareness to circulate the Pearl from the center of the palm to the tip of your middle finger and then back to the center again. Feel the Pearl trace a clear path. Keep the Pearl circulating back and forth along that path. Feel the energy pathway created by the Pearl becoming stronger and visualize it growing brighter. After a few cycles, relax your mind and allow the Pearl to glide up and down this pathway effortlessly like a pendulum swinging back and forth.

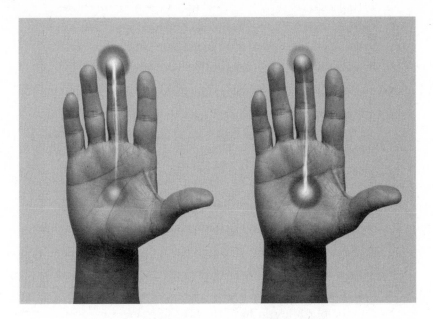

Figure 6.11: Circulating the Pearl

Next, circulate the Pearl from the center to the tip of your index finger and back. Repeat several times until you feel the Pearl gliding smoothly. Circulate the Pearl to your thumb and back. And then to the ring finger, and then the small finger. Take your time. Feel the energetic pathways of your hand open up and become more palpable.

In the rest of the exercise that follows, we systematize the process that we just used to make a Pearl. This time we will form a Pearl on your left hand.

1. Become aware of the center of your left palm.

2. Concentrate and use your intention in conjunction with your eye movement to trace a plus sign on your palm. Begin with the horizontal line, then the vertical. Repeat each line three times or more.

3. When you feel the plus sign clearly, trace a multiplication sign in the same way.

4. Become aware of the plus sign and the multiplication sign forming an eight-pointed Bagua star on your palm. Feel a heavy sensation on your palm. This is Palm Qi.

5. Trace a Taiji spiral from the edge of the Bagua star to the center point. Allow the spiral to concentrate Palm Qi at the center. As you reach the center point, concentrate the Palm Qi into a Pearl.

6. Feel the dense presence of a Pearl at the center of your palm.

7. Circulate the Pearl along a smooth line from the center of the palm to your middle fingertip, and then back to the center. Repeat several times.

8. Trace a smooth pathway to each of the fingertips and back to the center. Begin with the second finger, and then the thumb, fourth finger, and finally the fifth finger.

9. Bring the Pearl back to the center of your palm and nourish your Palm. *I am in Qi; Qi is in me.*

Awakening Baihui

Earlier, you circulated a Pearl between the center of your palm and your fingertips. If you surveyed a detailed acupuncture chart depicting the Meridians, you would not find Meridian lines covering those pathways. We created those pathways arbitrarily. If you wanted to form a Pearl at the tip of your nose, and to circulate that Pearl across your face to your earlobe and back, you could. You can create Pearls and energy lines connecting any two points on the body. The energy body is highly malleable. This is not to say that the traditional Meridian lines are arbitrary. Those lines are well established.

Think of a dry riverbed. Torrential rains would pour into the riverbed and follow its natural contours. But if we dug a trench that extended away from the riverbed, the waters would flow into it as well. Similarly, we can divert the flow of Qi of a Meridian line toward a specific point by creating that connection through our intention. Throughout this chapter we will be doing just that. Every Meridian line is going to be rerouted to arguably the most prominent Energy Point in the body, Baihui—the Energy Point that crowns the head.

To find Baihui, trace a line from your ears to the midpoint of your cranium. If you grazed your head on the lintel of a short door, you found Baihui. Baihui defines the summit of the cranium. As previously mentioned, Baihui is the physical analogue of Pure Mind, and the time has come to awaken it.

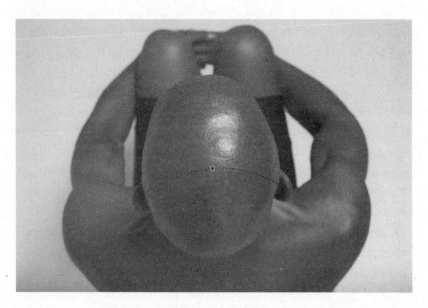

Figure 6.12: Baihui

Imagine asking every person on earth who believes in God to point toward heaven. Instinctively, the vast majority would point overhead toward the sky. Everyone would be pointing in a different direction since the earth is a sphere. But they would all be pointing in the same direction relative to the top of their head, Baihui. When Baihui is awakened, our sense of divinity and sacredness is activated. The more open and receptive Baihui is, the easier it is for us to experience a divine presence. What divinity? That depends on your religious belief. The form of the divine often reflects the cultural matrix into which we are born. But even someone who does not recognize any deity or religion will experience a sense of the sacred when Baihui is activated. When Baihui is awakened, we all experience a connection to something gloriously greater than ourselves, and we are humbled by the recognition of holiness.

The natural flow of the Meridian lines does not extend naturally to Baihui, but we will create those energetic connections just like we create a pathway between the center of our palm and our fingertips. The energetic "trenches" that we will be creating are going to divert all twelve Meridian lines to Baihui. Energy will flow from the Organs to Baihui. From Baihui to the fingertips and toes. Energy will flow from the fingertips and toes to Baihui. And from Baihui back to the Organs. Baihui is going to become the central hub of the Meridian network.

As we direct Organ Qi to Baihui, the quality of sacredness, divinity, and holiness is going to blend with the Organ Virtues—all of them. The kindness of the Lungs is going to blend with Baihui Qi, resulting in a more exalted virtue: Sacred Kindness. When you express Sacred Kindness, the person on the receiving end of your goodness feels blessed. When the courage of the Gallbladder blends with Baihui Qi, the exalted virtue of Sacred Courage is generated. When Baihui Qi blends with the qualities of the Twelve Meridians, the quality of sacredness spreads throughout the body to the very tips of your fingers and toes. Pure Mind is associated with Baihui, and when we integrate the Baihui Qi of Pure Mind and the Organ Qi of Higher Mind, our psyche becomes saturated with divine qualities. Experientially, when we integrate Organ Qi and Baihui, we feel blessed, and we feel like blessing those around us.

Exercise 28: Awakening Baihui

In this exercise, we awaken Baihui by forming a Pearl at the top of the head and resonating the chant of the Upper Dantian—Ong, *ongggg* . . . to further stimulate the point. We direct Ong to the top of the head. Then we whisper Ong to enter Baihui and heal Pure Mind. Finally, we mouth Ong to empower Baihui.

1. Adopt Natural Sitting Posture and practice Taiji Breathing for three cycles or more until your mind is calm.

2. Become aware of Baihui.

3. Form a Pearl at Baihui. Trace an eight-pointed star at the top of your head and then circulate a Taiji toward the center of the star. Concentrate the energy and form a Baihui Pearl.

4. Chant Ong, *ongggg* . . . the sound of the Upper Dantian. Direct the vibration from the center of your head to Baihui. Repeat three times or more.

5. Whisper Ong to heal Baihui. Feel your awareness sink into the Energy Point at the top of your head. Scan Baihui. Whisper Ong and release any negativity that arises. Repeat three times or more. Abide in the bliss of Baihui for as long as you please.

6. Mouth Ong to empower Baihui. Repeat three times or more.

7. If you are inspired to pray or bless someone, this is the time to do it.

8. Practice Taiji Breathing to focus Qi to your Lower Dantian.

9. Nourish your Qi. *I am in Qi; Qi is in me.*

Once Baihui is awakened and you can feel even just a spark of Sacred Qi emanating from the top of your head, you are ready to Bless the Organs.

Exercise 29: Blessing the Organs

This exercise develops a pathway between Baihui and each of the twelve Organs. We use chanting to awaken an Organ and Baihui, and then circulate energy between the two.

1. Adopt Natural Sitting Posture and practice Taiji Breathing for three cycles or more until your mind is calm.

2. Awaken your Lungs by chanting Si (*Szzzzz . . .*). And then awaken Baihui by chanting Ong. Inhale at Baihui and exhale Baihui Qi to the Lungs. Bless your Lungs. Inhale Lung Qi to Baihui. Abide in the benevolence of kindness. Repeat three or more times.

3. Awaken your Large Intestine by chanting Si (*Szzzzz . . .*). And then awaken Baihui by chanting Ong. Inhale at Baihui and exhale Baihui Qi to the Large Intestine. Bless your Large Intestine. Inhale Large Intestine Qi to Baihui. Abide in the benevolence of honesty. Repeat three or more times.

4. Awaken your Stomach by chanting Hu (*Whoooo . . .*). And then awaken Baihui by chanting Ong. Inhale at Baihui and exhale Baihui Qi to the Stomach. Bless your Stomach. Inhale Stomach Qi to Baihui. Abide in the benevolence of your satisfaction. Repeat three or more times.

5. Awaken your Spleen by chanting Hu (*Whoooo . . .*). And then awaken Baihui by chanting Ong. Inhale at Baihui and exhale Baihui Qi to the Spleen. Bless your Spleen. Inhale Spleen Qi to Baihui. Abide in the benevolence of your clarity. Repeat three or more times.

6. Awaken your Heart by chanting Ha (*Haaaaa . . .*). And then awaken Baihui by chanting Ong. Inhale at Baihui and exhale Baihui Qi to the Heart. Bless your Heart. Inhale Heart Qi to Baihui. Abide in the benevolence of your dignity. Repeat three or more times.

7. Awaken your Small Intestine by chanting Ha (*Haaaaa . . .*). And then awaken Baihui by chanting Ong. Inhale at Baihui and exhale Baihui Qi to the Small Intestine. Bless your Small Intestine. Inhale Small Intestine Qi to Baihui. Abide in the benevolence of your discernment. Repeat three or more times.

8. Awaken your Urinary Bladder by chanting Chui (*Chuwee . . .*). And then awaken Baihui by chanting Ong.

Inhale at Baihui and exhale Baihui Qi to the Urinary
Bladder. Bless your Urinary Bladder. Inhale Urinary Bladder
Qi to Baihui. Abide in the benevolence of your freedom.
Repeat three or more times.

9. Awaken your Kidneys by chanting Chui (*Chuwee . . .*). And
then awaken Baihui by chanting Ong. Inhale at Baihui and
exhale Baihui Qi to the Kidneys. Bless your Kidneys. Inhale
Kidneys Qi to Baihui. Abide in the benevolence of your
persistence. Repeat three or more times.

10. Awaken your Pericardium by chanting Xi (*Sheeee . . .*). And
then awaken Baihui by chanting Ong. Inhale at Baihui and
exhale Baihui Qi to the Pericardium. Bless your Pericardium.
Inhale Pericardium Qi to Baihui. Abide in the benevolence of
your caring nature. Repeat three or more times.

11. Awaken your San Jiao by chanting Xi (*Sheeee . . .*). And
then awaken Baihui by chanting Ong. Inhale at Baihui and
exhale Baihui Qi to the San Jiao. Bless your San Jiao. Inhale
San Jiao Qi to Baihui. Abide in the benevolence of your
coherence. Repeat three or more times.

12. Awaken your Gallbladder by chanting Xu (*Shewww . . .*).
And then awaken Baihui by chanting Ong. Inhale at
Baihui and exhale Baihui Qi to the Gallbladder. Bless your
Gallbladder. Inhale Gallbladder Qi to Baihui. Abide in the
benevolence of your courage. Repeat three or more times.

13. Awaken your Liver by chanting Xu (*Shewww . . .*). And then
awaken Baihui by chanting Ong. Inhale at Baihui and exhale
Baihui Qi to the Liver. Bless your Liver. Inhale Liver Qi to
Baihui. Abide in the benevolence of your enthusiasm. Repeat
three or more times.

14. Become aware of the sky. Become aware of Baihui. Become aware
of your internal Organs. Feel blessed and bless the Universe.

15. Practice Taiji Breathing to focus your Qi at the Lower Dantian.

16. Nourish your Qi. *I am in Qi; Qi is in me.*

The Meridian Clock

Perhaps you noticed that we are following a different sequence in this chapter than we followed with the Six Healing Sounds. With the Six Healing Sounds we began the exercises with the Liver Family, then the Heart Family, Spleen Family, Lung Family, Kidney Family, and finally the San Jiao Family. The sequence in this chapter begins with the Lung Family, then the Spleen Family, the Heart Family, Kidney Family, San Jiao Family, and finally the Liver Family.

The sequence that we follow in this chapter reflects the time frames of peak activity for the Organs over the course of the day. The notion is that at specific hours of the day, a particular Organ becomes more active. Just as certain activities are regulated seasonally, certain activities are regulated daily. There are twenty-four hours per day so that each one of the twelve Organs is assigned a two-hour peak period. During that period, a particular Organ and its Meridian are relatively more active as their functions are emphasized. When we align our daily activities with the *Meridian Clock*, we are following the natural order of energy flow and minimizing stress on the Organ system. When we deviate from the natural order, our Organs must work harder to keep up with the demands of the day.

The Meridian Clock is described below.

Lungs (3:00 am – 5:00 am)

Respiration is related to the production of Qi. The deeper we breathe, the slower we breathe, the more Qi we harvest from each breath. Since the Meridian Clock tracks the flow of Qi and the Lungs are most closely associated with the absorption of Qi in the form of air, the cycle begins with the Lungs. The time interval assigned to the Lungs coincides with the time of night when we are least likely to be talking and most likely to be breathing deeply. This is the peak time when Qi flows throughout the Lung Meridian with the greatest potency for nourishing the Lungs and healing the functions associated with the Lungs. If someone expends

Lung Qi between 3:00 am and 5:00 am by working those hours on a regular basis, their Lungs and their related qualities would be weakened.

Large Intestine (5:00 am – 7:00 am)

Most people wake up during this time interval. This is the ideal time to drink warm water to hydrate the Large Intestine and initiate a bowel movement. The elimination of waste is the function that is emphasized during this two-hour period. Letting go of toxic waste that no longer serves us reflects the function of Large Intestine Qi. The feeling of lightness after a morning bowel movement is the feeling of purgation associated with the Large Intestine.

Stomach (7:00 am – 9:00 am)

This is the time to eat a satisfying breakfast that will nourish the body. The hearty appetite of breakfast is the energy of a Stomach eager to accumulate food. The energy of satisfaction after eating a wholesome breakfast reflects the contentment and pleasure associated with Stomach Qi. If we follow our appetite and eat a nutritious breakfast, our energy level throughout the day remains high. If we eat an unwholesome breakfast, we feel bloated, weighed down, and less energetic throughout the day. The inborn intelligence of Stomach Qi directs our appetite toward the food most beneficial to our well-being. This intelligence becomes heightened during this two-hour interval.

Spleen (9:00 am – 11:00 am)

During this time interval, the food we ate for breakfast is being digested and we feel more energetic as our blood sugar level rises. The surge of energy that you experience as the morning waxes is indicative of Spleen Qi cresting. This is the right time for physical and mental activity. During this time, the body wants to move around and exercise. During this time, the mind is clearest. This is the ideal time to clarify your thoughts and think issues through. If you want to hold a meeting to explore new ideas, do it when the Meridian Clock points to the Spleen. Your cognitive abilities peak during this time.

Heart (11:00 am – 1:00 pm)

This is the time of the day when the sun peaks as well as the Heart. The Heart functions like a small sun providing the body with warmth and regulating circulation. During this time, our personal sense of power peaks. This time interval also coincides with lunchtime, when another surge of food energy courses through the body. This meal should be enjoyed and eaten in a cheerful atmosphere. Joy is a quality associated with Heart Qi. Rushing through lunch strains the Heart.

Small Intestine (1:00 pm – 3:00 pm)

The heavy meal eaten at lunch is digested and assimilated during this time. By this time, our mind is moving more slowly than it was in the morning. We feel more lethargic after eating lunch than after eating breakfast. While the Spleen time (9:00 am – 11:00 am) is ideal for exploratory work and jam sessions, Small Intestine time is more suited to performing menial tasks like sorting and organizing.

Urinary Bladder (3:00 pm – 5:00 pm)

Energetically, this is a good time to plan for tomorrow. Sipping a cup of tea while focusing on future plans and creating to-do lists are activities suited to this timeframe. This is the time to cast off heavy burdens and begin to unwind as we close out the workday. If we feel oppressed or limited in some way by a toxic person or situation, this is the ideal time to address the issue.

Kidney (5:00 pm – 7:00 pm)

This timeframe is ideal for releasing the stress of the workday and shifting awareness inwardly. If we feel depleted during this time, our Kidneys are letting us know that we are leading an imbalanced lifestyle. As we let go of work, we should ideally look forward to the evening ahead. If we are caught up during this time interval thinking about issues that make us feel pressured and generate fear, we are depleting our Kidney Qi. Kidney time is the time to release the day and to look forward to dinnertime and nighttime activities.

Pericardium (7:00 pm – 9:00 pm)

This time interval is ideal for family time. This is the time to connect with people you care for. Romantically, this is the ideal time to allow someone into your Heart. Let your friends know that you appreciate them. Tell your children that you love them. This is the time to express tenderness and to allow your vulnerability to shine through. By this time, the night sky is beautiful with the moon and the stars spread across the heavens. This is the time to indulge your imagination. Watching a heart-felt movie or reading a novel heals the Pericardium. The image of a warm fireside chat captures the essence of this timeframe. This period is also ideal for sexual activity and conceiving a child.

San Jiao (9:00 pm – 11:00 pm)

During this timeframe, the body begins to wane. We become sleepy. Our Organs are tired from a full day of mental, emotional, physical, and metabolic activity. The Organs are signaling that the time for sleep is nearing. The body wants to begin conserving energy in anticipation of the coming day. If you pick up a book during this timeframe and begin to doze off, your San Jiao Qi is doing its work. If you are highly animated and overly excited by the time this timeframe ends, your San Jiao Qi is not properly balanced. As we approach the nadir of night, we should be ready to surrender to sleep.

Gallbladder (11:00 pm – 1:00 am)

At midnight, deep below the earth, the sun is starting its journey back up. This timeframe signals the shift between diurnal Yin and Yang. Gallbladder Qi is the most assertive and courageous energy that we express, and this quality is regenerated while we sleep during this time. If we lack "guts" during the day, it could be in part because we are not getting deep rest during the time of the Gallbladder. To wake up energized and ready to roar, we should strive to be in a state of deep sleep at this time.

Liver (1:00 am – 3:00 am)

During this time, the Liver is cleansing our blood and regenerating Liver Qi, which manifests as enthusiasm and optimism throughout our waking hours. The doorway to Spirit opens and the deepest restorative and healing sleep occurs during this timeframe. Deep wisdom and revelatory insights are communicated to us as we plunge into deep slumber. Otherworldly knowledge and intuitive guidance are provided as well. The capacity to take an inspired leap of faith in the face of unfavorable odds is linked to the quality of our deep sleep during this time. The ability to confidently seize the moment during the day is indicative of healthy Liver Qi cultivated by resting the Liver during this time.

Exercise 30: Awakening the Lung Thumb Points

An energetic connection between Baihui and the Organs has been established. The sequence of the flow of Qi throughout the Meridian network has been described. Now comes the hard work—connecting the Meridians and Baihui. We are going to awaken the Meridians in the order of the Meridian Clock. Awakening all the hundreds of Meridian points is impractical and unnecessary for us to achieve our objective. By activating just a few strategic points, we can stimulate the entire Meridian. For each Meridian, we are going to awaken four of the major Energy Points on that channel. Some of the longer Leg Meridians require five Energy Points.

The process we followed to form a Pearl at the center of your palm, and to circulate that Pearl to your fingertip and back, is the same process we are going to follow now to awaken segments of the Meridian. We are going to form a Pearl at an Energy Point and circulate that Pearl from one Energy

Point to the next Energy Point, and then back. Then those segments are interlinked, and the Pearl is circulated along the entire Meridian.

Every Energy Point has a Chinese name as well as an English name. For example, Lung 11, the last point of the Lung Meridian, is known as *Shaoshang*, which means *Lesser Metal*. Neither Shaoshang, Lung 11, nor the Lesser Metal add value for our purposes, and memorizing dozens of names would soon become a tiresome task. To keep the process of awakening the Energy Points simple and manageable, we will name the points by referencing their location. Instead of using the name Lung 11 or Shaoshang, we simply reference the Lung Thumb Point. In fact, before diving into deep waters, we will do a practice run and awaken the right Lung Thumb Point by forming a Pearl there to review the process in detail. All the other Energy Points follow the same procedure, so that once you form a Pearl at one Energy Point, you can apply the process to all the other Energy Points.

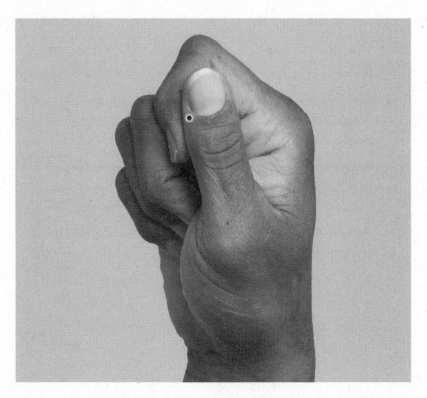

Figure 6.13: Lung Thumb Point

The right Lung Thumb Point is located near the lower inner corner of the nailbed on your right thumb. We awaken the Lung Thumb Point by forming a Pearl on that spot. We trace a Bagua and then spiral a Taiji toward the center until the Qi concentrates into a dense energy presence, a Pearl. Once we have awakened the Thumb Lung Point, we can create an instantaneous Lung Thumb Point Pearl. We simply bring our attention to the Energy Point and concentrate our attention on the center.

Once the Lung Thumb Point is awakened, we are going to integrate the Energy Point into the Lung Family. Begin by chanting the Lung Healing Sound, Si, *szzzzz* . . . and direct the resonance to the Lung Thumb Point. Next, we whisper Si at the Lung Thumb Point, and then we mouth Si at the Lung Thumb Point. Finally, we chant Si and feel the resonance vibrate the Nose, Lungs, Large Intestine, and the Lung Thumb Point.

The instructions that follow detail the steps used to integrate the Lung Thumb Point into the Lung Family.

Part 1: Form a Pearl

1. Become aware of the Lung Thumb Point on your right hand.

2. Create a Bagua centering on the right Lung Thumb Point. Trace a plus sign over the point. Use your eye movement to deepen the sensation: side to side and up and down.

3. Trace a multiplication sign over the point. Use your eye movement to deepen the sensation: a diagonal line and then a diagonal line.

4. Feel the eight-point Bagua star and spiral a Taiji toward the center of the Bagua.

5. As the energy concentrates, feel the Pearl form. Feel a dense and lingering presence at the point.

6. Repeat this process with the left Lung Thumb Point.

Part 2: Integrate the point into the Organ Family

7. Chant the Lung Family sound, Si: *Szzzzz* . . . Direct the resonance to the two Lung Thumb Points. Repeat three times or more.

8. Whisper Si to heal the Lung Thumb Points. Repeat three times or more.

9. Mouth Si to empower the Lung Thumb Points. Repeat three times or more.

10. Chant the Lung Family sound, Si, and direct the resonance to your Nose, Lungs, Large Intestine, and Lung Thumb Points. Repeat three times or more. The Lung Thumb Points are now integrated into the Lung Family.

11. Nourish the Qi of your expanded Lung Family. *I am in Qi; Qi is in me.*

Awakening the Twelve Meridians

We are now ready to awaken and empower the Meridians starting with the two Lung Meridians.

The Lung Meridian

The Qi flow of the Lung Meridian begins at the Lungs. We form a Pearl at the Lungs. The point where the Pearl is formed is located in the sternum where the bronchial tube divides into the right and left bronchi. If you take a strong breath through your nose, you can feel the point where the airflow splits. The Lung Qi Pearl is formed at that point. The Lung Qi Pearl is then inhaled up to Baihui and exhaled down to the Lung Shoulder Point, the Lung Elbow Point, the Lung Wrist Point, and finally to the Lung Thumb Point that we previously awakened. Previously, we also awakened the energy pathway between the Lungs and Baihui. Awakening the Lung Meridian requires a few additional steps:

1. We must awaken the four Energy points mentioned above on the right side and on the left side by forming Pearls at each point.

2. We circulate a Pearl back and forth between every two points to concentrate Qi along that segment of the Meridian. For example, we form a Pearl at the Lung Shoulder Point and circulate that Pearl to the Lung Elbow Point and then back to the Lung Shoulder Point. Cycling the Pearl between two points brings awareness to the part of the Meridian covered in that segment. We awaken the points on both sides of the body and then cycle the Pearl bilaterally.

3. Next, we chant, whisper, and mouth the Lung Sound, Si, and resonate the Lungs and the segment of the Meridian between the Lung Shoulder Point and the Lung Thumb Point. This process integrates the Energy Points and the Lung Meridian into the Lung Family. We repeat the process on the left side.

4. Finally, we integrate the Lungs, Baihui, and the two Meridians by chanting Si. This process integrates Higher Mind and Pure Mind, drawing together the Organ Virtue of the Lungs and Baihui Qi.

The illustration below depicts Qi flow from the Lungs to Baihui and along the two Lung Meridians. The instructions for the exercise follow below.

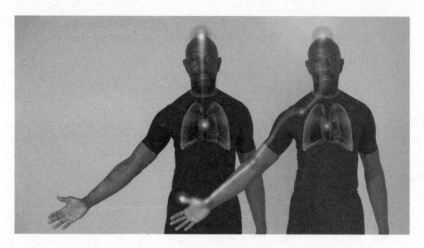

Figure 6.14: Lung Meridian

Lung Meridian	Location	Traditional Name
1. Lungs	Upper thoracic cavity	
2. Baihui	Crown	GV 20
3. Lung Shoulder Point	Depression in shoulder next to clavicle	LU 2, Yunmen
4. Lung Elbow Point	Elbow crease on Lung line	LU 5, Chize
5. Lung Wrist Point	Wrist crease on Lung line	LU 9, Taiyuan
6. Lung Finger Point	Radial side, thumb nailbed	LU 11, Shaoshang

Exercise 31: Empower the Lung Meridians

Part 1: Awaken the Lung Shoulder Point

1. Become aware of the right Lung Shoulder Point.

2. Form a Pearl at the Lung Shoulder Point.

3. Chant the Lung Sound, Si. Feel the Lung Family and the point resonate as you chant. Integrate the point into the Lung Family. Repeat three times or more.

4. Awaken the Left Lung Shoulder Point using the same procedure.

Part 2: Awaken the rest of the Lung Energy Points

5. Repeat part 1 with the Lung Elbow Points.

6. Repeat part 1 with the Lung Wrist Points.

7. Repeat part 1 with the Lung Thumb Points.

8. Repeat part 1 and form a Lung Qi Pearl at the end of the bronchial tube between the Lungs.

Part 3: Circulate the Lung Meridian Pearl

9. Become aware of your Lungs. Form a Lung Qi Pearl. Inhale the Lung Qi Pearl to Baihui.

10. Exhale the Pearl from Baihui to the right Lung Shoulder Point, and inhale it back to Baihui. Cycle the Pearl back and forth until that section of the Meridian becomes palpable.

11. Exhale the Pearl from the Lung Shoulder Point to the Lung Elbow Point, and inhale it back. Cycle the Pearl back and forth until that section of the Meridian becomes palpable.

12. Exhale the Pearl from the right Lung Elbow Point to the Lung Wrist Point, and inhale it back. Cycle the Pearl back and forth until the pathway becomes clear, and awareness of that section of the Meridian becomes palpable.

13. Exhale the Pearl from the right Lung Wrist Point to the Lung Finger Point, and inhale it back. Cycle the energy back and forth until that section of the Meridian becomes palpable.

14. Repeat part 3 on the left side.

Part 4: Empower the Lung Meridians

15. Become aware of the Lungs and form a Lung Qi Pearl. Inhale the Lung Qi Pearl to Baihui.

16. As you exhale, chant Si, *szzzzz* . . . Feel the vibration travel from Baihui along the right Lung Meridian to the Lung Thumb Point. Repeat three times or more.

17. Abide in the Qi flow of your Lung Meridian. Feel the quality of benevolence flowing through your Lung Meridian. Awaken and bless your Lung Meridian.

18. Repeat part 4 on the left side.

Part 5: Integrate the two Meridians

19. Inhale the Lung Qi Pearl to Baihui, chant Si, *szzzzz* . . . and circulate two Pearls at the same time from Baihui along both Lung Meridians to the Lung Thumb Points. Feel the quality of benevolence flowing though both Lung Meridians. Repeat three or more times.

20. Nourish your Qi. *I am in Qi; Qi is in me.*

The Large Intestine Meridian

The Qi flow of the Large Intestine Meridian begins at the Large Intestine Finger Point. We inhale up from that point to the Large Intestine Wrist Point, the Large Intestine Elbow Point, the Large Intestine Shoulder Point, up to Baihui, and then we exhale the Pearl down to the Large Intestine, specifically to the anus.

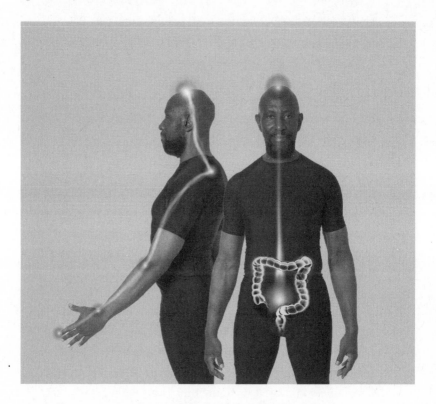

Figure 6.15: Large Intestine Meridian

Large Intestine Meridian	Location	Traditional Name
1. Large Intestine Finger Point	Radial side, second finger nailbed	LI 1, Shangyang
2. Large Intestine Wrist Point	Wrist depression on large intestine line	LI 5, Yangxi
3. Large Intestine Elbow Point	Flex elbow ninety degrees. Depression between the elbow crease and the bone.	LI 11, Quchi
4. Large Intestine Shoulder Point	Depression between outer prominence of scapula and the spine of scapula	LI 16, Jugu
5. Baihui	Crown	GV 20
6. Large Intestine	Lower abdominal cavity	

Exercise 32: Empower the Large Intestine Meridians

Part 1: Awaken the Large Intestine Finger Point

1. Become aware of the right Large Intestine Finger Point.

2. Form a Pearl at the Large Intestine Finger Point.

3. Chant the Large Intestine Family Sound, Hu. Feel the Lung Family and the point resonate as you chant. Integrate the point into the Lung Family. Repeat three times or more.

4. Repeat part 1 on the left side.

Part 2: Awaken the Rest of the Large Intestine Energy Points

5. Repeat part 1 with the Large Intestine Wrist Points.

6. Repeat part 1 with the Large Intestine Elbow Points.

7. Repeat part 1 with the Large Intestine Shoulder Points.

Part 3: Circulate the Large Intestine Meridian Pearl

8. Become aware of your right Large Intestine Finger Point. Inhale and form a Pearl at the Large Intestine Finger Point, and exhale the Pearl to the Large Intestine Wrist Point. Cycle the Pearl back and forth until that section of the Meridian becomes palpable.

9. Inhale the Pearl at the Large Intestine Wrist Point, and exhale it to the Large Intestine Elbow Point and back. Cycle the Pearl back and forth until that section of the Meridian becomes palpable.

10. Inhale the Pearl at the Large Intestine Elbow Point, and exhale it to the Large Intestine Shoulder Point and back. Cycle the Pearl back and forth until that section of the Meridian becomes palpable.

11. Inhale the Pearl at the Large Intestine Shoulder Point, and exhale to Baihui, and inhale it back. Cycle the Pearl back and forth until that section of the Meridian becomes palpable.

12. Inhale the Pearl at Baihui, and exhale Baihui Qi to the anus at the end of the Large Intestine. Cycle the energy back and forth until that section of the Meridian becomes palpable.

13. Repeat part 3 on the left side.

Part 4: Empower the Large Intestine Meridians

14. Become aware of the right Large Intestine Finger Point and form a Pearl. Inhale the Pearl along the right Large Intestine Meridian to Baihui.

15. As you exhale, chant Si, *szzzzz* . . . Feel the vibration travel from Baihui to the anus at the end of the Large Intestine. Repeat three times or more.

16. Abide in your Large Intestine. Feel the quality of benevolence in your Large Intestine. Awaken and bless your Large Intestine.

17. Repeat part 4 on the left side.

Part 5: Integrate the two Meridians

18. Inhale two Pearls from both Large Intestine Finger Points along the Large Intestine Meridians to Baihui. Chant Si, *szzzzz* . . . as you direct the Pearl to the anus at the end of the Large Intestine. Feel the quality of benevolence in your Large Intestine. Repeat three or more times.

19. Nourish your Qi. *I am in Qi; Qi is in me.*

The Stomach Meridian

The Stomach Meridian begins at the stomach. A Stomach Qi Pearl is formed at the center of the Stomach and inhaled up to Baihui and exhaled down to the Navel, Stomach Hip Point, Stomach Knee Point, Stomach Ankle Point, and finally to the Stomach Toe Point.

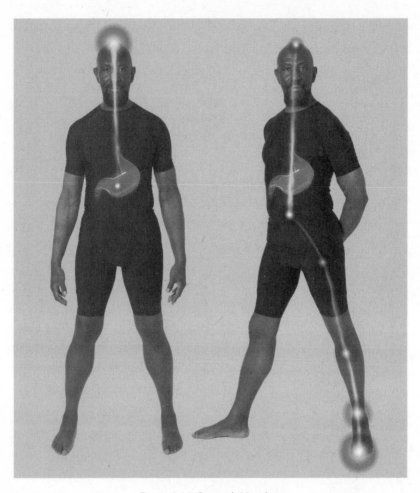

Figure 6.16: Stomach Meridian

Stomach Meridian	Location	Traditional Name
1. Stomach	Beneath liver on right side	
2. Baihui	Crown	GV 20
3. Navel	Navel	CV 8, Shenque
4. Stomach Hip Point	In a depression at the bottom of hip bone prominence in line with the pubic bone	ST 31, Biguan
5. Stomach Knee Point	One finger width lateral to the crest of the leg bone	ST 36, Zusanli
6. Stomach Ankle Point	In a depression in the front of the ankle in line with the ankle bone	ST 41, Jiexi
7. Stomach Toe Point	Lateral side, second toe nailbed	ST 45, Lidui

Exercise 33: Empower the Stomach Meridians

Part 1: Awaken the Navel

1. Become aware of the Navel.

2. Form a Pearl at the Navel.

3. Chant the Spleen Family Sound, Hu. Feel the Spleen Family and the point resonate as you chant. Integrate the point into the Spleen Family. Repeat three times or more.

Part 2: Awaken the Rest of the Stomach Energy Points

4. Repeat part 1 with the Stomach Hip Points.

5. Repeat part 1 with the Stomach Knee Points.

6. Repeat part 1 with the Stomach Ankle Points.

7. Repeat part 1 with the Stomach Toe Points.

8. Repeat part 1 and create a Stomach Qi Pearl at the center of your Stomach.

Part 3: Circulate the Stomach Meridian Pearl

9. Become aware of your Stomach. Inhale a Stomach Qi Pearl to Baihui at the top of your head.

10. Exhale the Pearl to the Navel, and inhale it back to Baihui. Cycle the Pearl back and forth until that section of the Meridian becomes palpable.

11. Exhale the Pearl from the Navel to the right Stomach Hip Point, and inhale it back. Cycle the Pearl back and forth until that section of the Meridian becomes palpable.

12. Exhale the Pearl from the right Stomach Hip Point to the right Stomach Knee Point, and inhale it back. Cycle the Pearl back and forth until the pathway becomes clear and awareness of that section of the Meridian becomes palpable.

13. Exhale the Pearl from the right Stomach Knee Point to the right Stomach Ankle Point, and inhale it back. Cycle the energy back and forth until that section of the Meridian becomes palpable.

14. Exhale the Pearl from the right Stomach Ankle Point to the right Stomach Toe Point, and inhale it back. Cycle the energy back and forth until that section of the Meridian becomes palpable.

15. Repeat part 3 on the left side.

Part 4: Empower the Stomach Meridians

16. Become aware of the Stomach. Inhale a Stomach Qi Pearl to Baihui.

17. As you exhale, chant Hu, *whoooo* . . . Feel the vibration travel from Baihui along the right Stomach Meridian to the right Stomach Toe Point. Repeat three times or more.

18. Abide in the Qi flow of your Stomach Meridian. Feel the quality of benevolence flowing through your Stomach Meridian. Awaken and bless your Stomach Meridian.

19. Repeat part 4 on the left side.

Part 5: Integrate the Two Meridians

20. Inhale a Stomach Qi Pearl to Baihui, chant Hu, *whoooo* . . . and circulate two Pearls at the same time from Baihui along both Stomach Meridians to the Stomach Toe Points. Feel the quality of benevolence flowing though both Stomach Meridians. Repeat three or more times.

21. Nourish your Qi. *I am in Qi; Qi is in me.*

The Spleen Meridian

The Spleen Meridian begins at the Spleen Toe Point. We inhale up from that point to the Spleen Ankle Point, the Spleen Knee Point, the Spleen Hip Point, the Navel, up to Baihui, and then we exhale the energy down to the center of the Spleen.

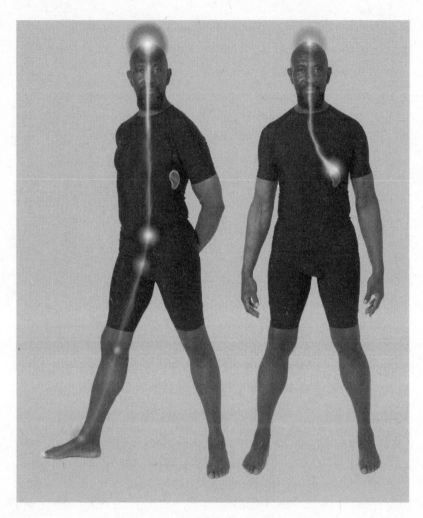

Figure 6.17: Spleen Meridian

Spleen Meridian	Location	Traditional Name
1. Spleen Toe Point	Medial side, first toe nailbed	SP 1, Yinbai
2. Spleen Ankle Point	Depression beside the front lower corner of inner ankle bone	SP 5, Shangqiu
3. Spleen Knee Point	In a depression below the end of the inner part of the thigh bone	SP 9, Yinlingquan
4. Spleen Hip Point	Find the top of the pubic bone. Move three to four inches to the side. Find the sensitive point in that area.	SP 12, Chongmen
5. Navel	Belly button	CV 8, Shenque
6. Baihui	Crown	GV 20
7. Spleen	Below diaphragm, posterior to liver and spleen	

Exercise 34: Empower the Spleen Meridians

Part 1: Awaken the Spleen Toe Point

1. Become aware of the right Spleen Toe Point.

2. Form a Pearl at the right Spleen Toe Point.

3. Chant the Spleen Family Sound, Chui. Feel the Spleen Family and the point resonate as you chant. Integrate the point into the Spleen Family. Repeat three times or more.

4. Repeat part 1 on the left side.

Part 2: Awaken the Rest of the Spleen Energy Points

5. Repeat part 1 with the Spleen Ankle Points.

6. Repeat part 1 with the Spleen Knee Points.

7. Repeat part 1 with the Spleen Hip Points.

8. Repeat part 1 with the Navel.

9. Repeat part 1 at the center of the Spleen.

Part 3: Circulate the Spleen Meridian Pearl

10. Become aware of your right Spleen Toe Point. Inhale and form a Pearl at the right Spleen Toe Point, and exhale the Pearl to the right Spleen Ankle Point. Cycle the Pearl back and forth until that section of the Meridian becomes palpable.

11. Inhale the Pearl at the right Spleen Ankle Point, and exhale it to the right Spleen Knee Point and back. Cycle the Pearl back and forth until that section of the Meridian becomes palpable.

12. Inhale the Pearl at the right Spleen Knee Point, and exhale it to the right Spleen Hip Point and back. Cycle the Pearl back and forth until that section of the Meridian becomes palpable.

13. Inhale the Pearl at the right Spleen Hip Point, and exhale it to the Navel and back. Cycle the Pearl back and forth until that section of the Meridian becomes palpable.

14. Inhale the Pearl at the Navel, and exhale it to Baihui, and inhale it back. Cycle the Pearl back and forth until that section of the Meridian becomes palpable.

15. Inhale the Pearl at Baihui, and exhale Baihui Qi to the center of the Spleen. Cycle the energy back and forth until that section of the Meridian becomes palpable.

16. Repeat part 3 on the left side.

Part 4: Empower the Spleen Meridians

17. Become aware of the right Spleen Toe Point and form a Pearl. Inhale the Pearl along the right Spleen Meridian to Baihui.

18. As you exhale, chant Hu, *whoooo* . . . Feel the vibration travel from Baihui to the Spleen. Repeat three times or more.

19. Abide in your Spleen. Feel the quality of benevolence in your Spleen. Awaken and bless your Spleen.

20. Repeat part 4 on the left side.

Part 5: Integrate the two Meridians

21. Inhale two Pearls from both Spleen Toe Points up the Spleen Meridians to Baihui. Chant Hu, *whoooo* . . . as you direct the Pearl to the center of the Spleen. Feel the quality of benevolence in your Spleen. Repeat three or more times.

22. Nourish your Qi. *I am in Qi; Qi is in me.*

The Heart Meridian

The Heart Meridian begins at the center of the Heart. A Heart Qi Pearl is inhaled up to Baihui and exhaled down to the Heart Shoulder Point, the Heart Elbow Point, the Heart Wrist Point, and finally to the Heart Finger Point.

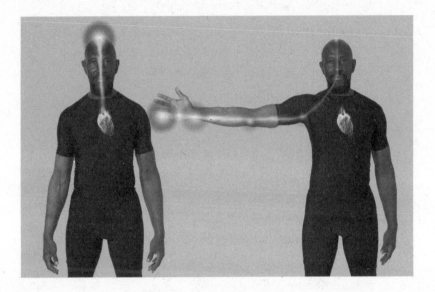

Figure 6.18: Heart Meridian

Heart Meridian	Location	Traditional Name
1. Heart	Left thoracic cavity	
2. Baihui	Crown	GV 20
3. Heart Armpit Point	Center of armpit	HT 1, Jiquan
4. Heart Elbow Point	Elbow crease on heart line	HT 3, Shaohai
5. Heart Wrist Point	Wrist crease on heart line	HT 7, Shenmen
6. Heart Finger Point	Radial side, fifth finger nailbed	HT 9, Shaochong

Exercise 35: Empower the Heart Meridians

Part 1: Awaken the Heart Armpit Point

1. Become aware of the right Heart Armpit Point.

2. Form a Pearl at the right Heart Armpit Point.

3. Chant the Heart Sound, Ha. Feel the Heart Family and the point resonate as you chant. Integrate the point into the Heart Family. Repeat three times or more.

4. Awaken the left Heart Point using the same procedure.

Part 2: Awaken the rest of the Heart Energy Points

5. Repeat part 1 with the Heart Elbow Points.

6. Repeat part 1 with the Heart Wrist Points.

7. Repeat part 1 with the Heart Finger Points.

8. Gently repeat part 1 at the center of the Heart.

Part 3: Circulate the Heart Meridian Pearl

9. Become aware of your Heart. Form a Heart Qi Pearl at the center of the Heart and inhale the Pearl to Baihui.

10. Exhale the Pearl to the right Heart Armpit Point, and inhale it back to Baihui. Cycle the Pearl back and forth until that section of the Meridian becomes palpable.

11. Exhale the Pearl from the Heart Armpit Point to the right Heart Elbow Point, and inhale it back. Cycle the Pearl back and forth until that section of the Meridian becomes palpable.

12. Exhale the Pearl from the right Heart Elbow Point to the right Heart Wrist Point, and inhale it back. Cycle the Pearl back and forth until the pathway becomes clear and awareness of that section of the Meridian becomes palpable.

13. Exhale the Pearl from the right Heart Wrist Point to the Heart Finger Point, and inhale it back. Cycle the energy back and forth until that section of the Meridian becomes palpable.

14. Repeat part 3 on the left side.

Part 4: Empower the Heart Meridians

15. Become aware of the Heart. Inhale a Heart Qi Pearl to Baihui.

16. As you exhale, chant Ha, *haaaaa* . . . Feel the vibration travel from Baihui along the right Heart Meridian to the right Heart Finger Point. Repeat three times or more.

17. Abide in the Qi flow of your Heart Meridian. Feel the quality of benevolence flowing through your Heart Meridian. Awaken and bless your Heart Meridian.

18. Repeat part 4 on the left side.

Part 5: Integrate the two Meridians

19. Inhale the Heart Qi Pearl to Baihui, chant Ha, *haaaaa* . . . and circulate two Pearls at the same time from Baihui along both Heart Meridians to the Heart Finger Points. Feel the quality of benevolence flowing though both Heart Meridians. Repeat three or more times.

20. Nourish your Qi. *I am in Qi; Qi is in me.*

The Small Intestine Meridian

The Small Intestine Meridian begins at the Small Intestine Finger Point. We inhale up from that point to the Small Intestine Wrist Point, the Small Intestine Elbow Point, and the Small Intestine Shoulder Point, up to Baihui, and then we exhale the energy down to the center of the Small Intestine.

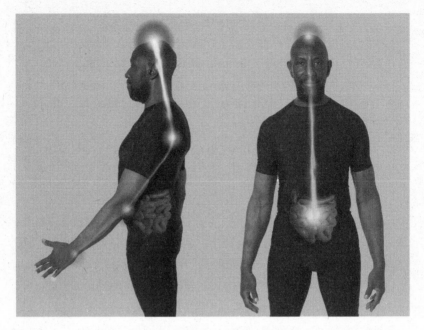

Figure 6.19: Small Intestine Meridian

Small Intestine Meridian	Location	Traditional Name
1. Small Intestine Finger Point	Ulnar side, fifth finger nailbed	SI 1, Shaoze
2. Small Intestine Wrist Point	Wrist depression on San Jiao line	SI 5, Yangu
3. Small Intestine Elbow Point	Flex elbow ninety degrees. Depression behind elbow tip.	SI 8, Xiaohai
4. Small Intestine Shoulder Point	Depression under the outermost part of the spine of shoulder blade	SI 9, Jianzhen
5. Baihui	Crown	GV 20
6. Small Intestine	Lower abdominal cavity under the stomach	

Exercise 36: Empower the Small Intestine Meridians

Part 1: Awaken the Small Intestine Finger Point

1. Become aware of the right Small Intestine Finger Point.

2. Form a Pearl at the right Small Intestine Finger Point.

3. Chant the Small Intestine Family Sound, Hu. Feel the Heart Family and the point resonate as you chant. Integrate the point into the Heart Family. Repeat three times or more.

4. Repeat part 1 on the left side.

Part 2: Awaken the Rest of the Small Intestine Energy Points

5. Repeat part 1 with the Small Intestine Wrist Points.

6. Repeat part 1 with the Small Intestine Elbow Points.

7. Repeat part 1 with the Small Intestine Shoulder Points.

8. Repeat part 1 at the center of the Small Intestine.

Part 3: Circulate the Small Intestine Meridian Pearl

9. Become aware of your right Small Intestine Finger Point. Inhale and form a Pearl at the right Small Intestine Finger Point, and exhale the Pearl to the right Small Intestine Wrist Point. Cycle the Pearl back and forth until that section of the Meridian becomes palpable.

10. Inhale the Pearl at the right Small Intestine Wrist Point, and exhale it to the right Small Intestine Elbow Point and back. Cycle the Pearl back and forth until that section of the Meridian becomes palpable.

11. Inhale the Pearl at the right Small Intestine Elbow Point, and exhale it to the right Small Intestine Shoulder Point and back. Cycle the Pearl back and forth until that section of the Meridian becomes palpable.

12. Inhale the Pearl at the right Small Intestine Shoulder Point, and exhale to Baihui and inhale it back. Cycle the Pearl back and forth until that section of the Meridian becomes palpable.

13. Inhale the Pearl at Baihui, and exhale Baihui Qi to the center of the Small Intestine. Cycle the energy back and forth until that section of the Meridian becomes palpable.

14. Repeat part 3 on the left side.

Part 4: Empower the Small Intestine Meridians

15. Become aware of the right Small Intestine Finger Point and form a Pearl. Inhale the Pearl along the right Small Intestine Meridian to Baihui.

16. As you exhale, chant Ha, *haaaaa . . .* Feel the vibration travel from Baihui to the Small Intestine. Repeat three times or more.

17. Abide in your Small Intestine. Feel the quality of benevolence in your Small Intestine. Awaken and bless your Small Intestine.

18. Repeat part 4 on the left side.

Part 5: Integrate the Two Meridians

19. Inhale two Pearls from both Small Intestine Finger Points along the Small Intestine Meridians to Baihui. Chant Ha, *haaaaa . . .* as you direct the Pearl to the center of the Small Intestine. Feel the quality of benevolence in your Small Intestine. Repeat three or more times.

20. Nourish your Qi. *I am in Qi; Qi is in me.*

The Urinary Bladder Meridian

The Urinary Bladder Meridian begins at the Urinary Bladder. A Urinary Bladder Qi Pearl is inhaled up to Baihui and exhaled down to the Tailbone Point, the Urinary Bladder Knee Point, the Urinary Bladder Ankle Point, and finally to the Urinary Bladder Toe Point.

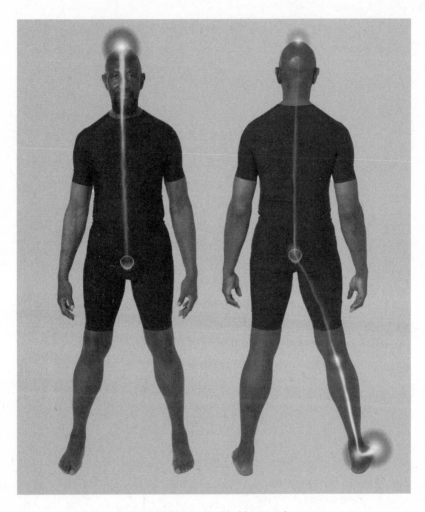

Figure 6.20: Urinary Bladder Meridian

Urinary Bladder Meridian	Location	Traditional Name
1. Urinary Bladder	Left thoracic cavity	
2. Baihui	Crown	GV 20
3. Tailbone Point	Tip of tailbone	UB 35, Huiyang
4. Urinary Bladder Knee Point	Midpoint of the knee crease	UB 40, Weizhong
5. Urinary Bladder Ankle Point	Depression between ankle bone and Achilles tendon	UB 60, Kunlun
6. Urinary Bladder Toe Point	Radial side, fifth finger nailbed	UB 67, Zhiyin

Exercise 37: Empower the Urinary Bladder Meridians

Part 1: Awaken the Tailbone Point

1. Become aware of the Tailbone Point.

2. Form a Pearl at the Tailbone Point.

3. Chant the Kidney Family Sound, Chui. Feel the Kidney Family and the point resonate as you chant. Integrate the point into the Kidney Family. Repeat three times or more.

Part 2: Awaken the Rest of the
Urinary Bladder Energy Points

4. Repeat part 1 with the Urinary Bladder Knee Points.

5. Repeat part 1 with the Urinary Bladder Ankle Points.

6. Repeat part 1 with the Urinary Bladder Toe Points.

7. Repeat part 1 at the center of the Urinary Bladder, where you experience the urge to urinate.

Part 3: Circulate the Urinary Bladder Meridian Pearl

8. Become aware of your Urinary Bladder. Inhale a Urinary Bladder Qi Pearl to Baihui at the top of your head.

9. Exhale the Pearl to the Tailbone Point, and inhale it back to Baihui. Cycle the Pearl back and forth until that section of the Meridian becomes palpable.

10. Exhale the Pearl from the Tailbone to the right Urinary Bladder Knee Point, and inhale it back. Cycle the Pearl back and forth until that section of the Meridian becomes palpable.

11. Exhale the Pearl from the right Urinary Bladder Knee Point to the right Urinary Bladder Ankle Point, and inhale it back. Cycle the energy back and forth until that section of the Meridian becomes palpable.

12. Exhale the Pearl from the right Urinary Bladder Ankle Point to the right Urinary Bladder Toe Point, and inhale it back. Cycle the energy back and forth until that section of the Meridian becomes palpable.

13. Repeat part 3 on the left side.

Part 4: Empower the Urinary Bladder Meridians

14. Become aware of the Urinary Bladder. Inhale a Urinary Bladder Qi Pearl to Baihui.

15. As you exhale, chant Hu, *whoooo* . . . Feel the vibration travel from Baihui along the right Urinary Bladder Meridian to the right Urinary Bladder Toe Point. Repeat three times or more.

16. Abide in the Qi flow of your Urinary Bladder Meridian. Feel the quality of benevolence flowing through your Urinary Bladder Meridian. Awaken and bless your Urinary Bladder Meridian.

17. Repeat part 4 on the left side.

Part 5: Integrate the Two Meridians

18. Inhale a Urinary Bladder Qi Pearl to Baihui, chant Hu, *whoooo* . . . and circulate two Pearls at the same time from Baihui along both Urinary Bladder Meridians to the Urinary Bladder Toe Points. Feel the quality of benevolence flowing though both Urinary Bladder Meridians. Repeat three or more times.

19. Nourish your Qi. *I am in Qi; Qi is in me.*

The Kidney Meridian

The Kidney Meridian begins at the Kidney Foot Point on the sole of the foot. From there, Qi is inhaled to the Kidney Ankle Point, the Kidney Knee Point, Huiyin at the perineum, up to Baihui, and then exhaled down to the center of each Kidney.

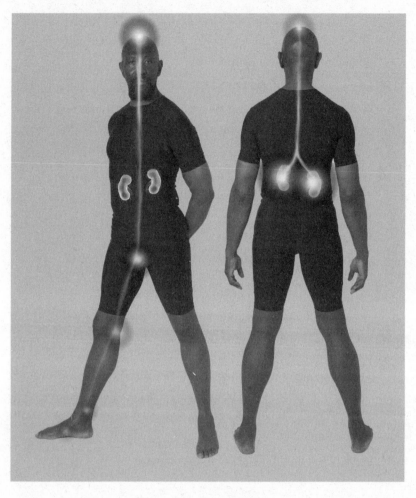

Figure 6.21: Kidney Meridian

Kidney Meridian	Location	Traditional Name
1. Kidney Foot Point	Crease of the foot when toes are extended	KI 1, Yongquan
2. Kidney Ankle Point	Sensitive point on the inside border of the Achilles tendon about two inches above the ankle	KI 7, Fuliu
3. Kidney Knee Point	With the knee bent ninety degrees, at the edge of the crease between the two hamstring tendons	KI 10, Yingu
4. Huiyin	Perineum, midway between anus and genitals	CV 1, Huiyin
5. Baihui	Crown	GV 20
6. Kidneys	Below diaphragm, posterior to liver and spleen	

Exercise 38: Empower the Kidney Meridians

Part 1: Awaken the Kidney Foot Point

1. Become aware of the right Kidney Foot Point.

2. Form a Pearl at the right Kidney Foot Point.

3. Chant the Kidney Family Sound, Chui. Feel the Kidney Family and the point resonate as you chant. Integrate the point into the Kidney Family. Repeat three times or more.

4. Repeat part 1 on the left side.

Part 2: Awaken the Rest of the Kidney Energy Points

5. Repeat part 1 with the Kidney Ankle Points.

6. Repeat part 1 with the Kidney Knee Points.

7. Repeat part 1 with Huiyin.

8. Repeat part 1 at the center of each Kidney.

Part 3: Circulate the Kidney Meridian Pearl

9. Become aware of your right Kidney Foot Point. Inhale and form a Pearl at the right Kidney Foot Point, and exhale the Pearl to the right Kidney Ankle Point. Cycle the Pearl back and forth until that section of the Meridian becomes palpable.

10. Inhale the Pearl at the right Kidney Ankle Point, and exhale it to the right Kidney Knee Point and back. Cycle the Pearl back and forth until that section of the Meridian becomes palpable.

11. Inhale the Pearl at the right Kidney Knee Point, and exhale it to Huiyin and back. Cycle the Pearl back and forth until that section of the Meridian becomes palpable.

12. Inhale the Pearl at Huiyin, and exhale it to Baihui, and inhale it back. Cycle the Pearl back and forth until that section of the Meridian becomes palpable.

13. Inhale the Pearl at Baihui, and exhale Baihui Qi to the center of each Kidney. Cycle the energy back and forth until that section of the Meridian becomes palpable.

14. Repeat part 3 on the left side.

Part 4: Empower the Kidney Meridians

15. Become aware of the right Kidney Foot Point and form a Pearl. Inhale the Pearl along the right Kidney Meridian to Baihui.

16. As you exhale, chant Chui, *chuwee* . . . Feel the vibration travel from Baihui to the Kidneys. Repeat three times or more.

17. Abide in your Kidneys. Feel the quality of benevolence in your Kidneys. Awaken and bless your Kidneys.

18. Repeat part 4 on the left side.

Part 5: Integrate the Two Meridians

19. Inhale two Pearls from both Kidney Toe Points up the Kidney Meridians to Baihui. Chant Chui, *chuwee* . . . as you direct the Pearl to the Kidneys. Feel the quality of benevolence in your Kidneys. Repeat three or more times.

20. Nourish your Qi. *I am in Qi; Qi is in me.*

The Pericardium Meridian

The Pericardium Meridian begins at the Pericardium. A Pericardium Qi Pearl is formed in the area around the Heart. The Pearl is inhaled up to Baihui and exhaled down to the Pericardium Shoulder Point, the Pericardium Elbow Point, the Pericardium Wrist Point, and finally to the Pericardium Finger Point.

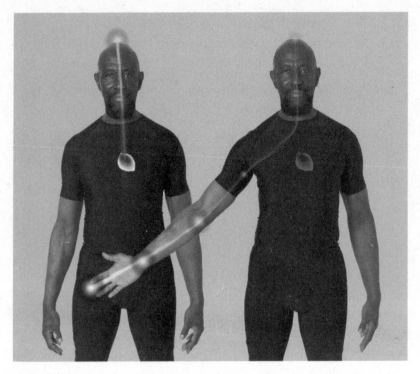

Figure 6.22: Pericardium Meridian

Pericardium Meridian	Location	Traditional Name
1. Pericardium	Membrane around the heart	
2. Baihui	Crown	GV 20
3. Pericardium Shoulder Point	A few inches below the ancillary fold where the two tendons of the bicep meet	PC 2, Tianquan
4. Pericardium Elbow Point	Elbow crease on pericardium line	PC 3, Quze
5. Pericardium Wrist Point	Wrist crease on pericardium line	PC 7, Daling
6. Pericardium Finger Point	Tip of the middle finger	PC 9, Zhongchong

Exercise 39: Empower the Pericardium Meridians

Part 1: Awaken the Pericardium Shoulder Point

1. Become aware of the right Pericardium Shoulder Point.

2. Form a Pearl at the right Pericardium Shoulder Point.

3. Chant the Pericardium Sound, Xi. Feel the San Jiao Family and the point resonate as you chant. Integrate the point into the San Jiao Family. Repeat three times or more.

4. Awaken the left Pericardium Point using the same procedure.

Part 2: Awaken the Rest of the
Pericardium Energy Points

5. Repeat part 1 with the Pericardium Elbow Points.

6. Repeat part 1 with the Pericardium Wrist Points.

7. Repeat part 1 with the Pericardium Finger Points.

8. Repeat part 1 at the Pericardium in the area around the Heart.

Part 3: Circulate the Pericardium Meridian Pearl

9. Become aware of your Pericardium. Inhale a Pericardium Qi Pearl to Baihui at the top of your head.

10. Exhale the Pearl to the right Pericardium Shoulder Point, and inhale it back to Baihui. Cycle the Pearl back and forth until that section of the Meridian becomes palpable.

11. Exhale the Pearl from the right Pericardium Shoulder Point to the right Pericardium Elbow Point, and inhale it back. Cycle the Pearl back and forth until that section of the Meridian becomes palpable.

12. Exhale the Pearl from the right Pericardium Elbow Point to the right Pericardium Wrist Point, and inhale it back. Cycle the Pearl back and forth until the pathway becomes clear and awareness of that section of the Meridian becomes palpable.

13. Exhale the Pearl from the right Pericardium Wrist Point to the right Pericardium Finger Point, and inhale it back. Cycle the energy back and forth until that section of the Meridian becomes palpable.

14. Repeat part 3 on the left side.

Part 4: Empower the Pericardium Meridians

15. Become aware of the Pericardium. Inhale a Pericardium Qi Pearl to Baihui.

16. As you exhale, chant Xi, *sheeee* . . . Feel the vibration travel from Baihui along the right Pericardium Meridian to the right Pericardium Finger Point. Repeat three times or more.

17. Abide in the Qi flow of your Pericardium Meridian. Feel the quality of benevolence flowing through your Pericardium Meridian. Awaken and bless your Pericardium Meridian.

18. Repeat part 4 on the left side.

Part 5: Integrate the Two Meridians

19. Inhale a Pericardium Qi Pearl to Baihui, chant Si, *sheeee* . . . and circulate two Pearls at the same time from Baihui along both Pericardium Meridians to the Pericardium Finger Points. Feel the quality of benevolence flowing though both Pericardium Meridians. Repeat three or more times.

20. Nourish your Qi. *I am in Qi; Qi is in me.*

The San Jiao Meridian

The San Jiao Meridian begins at the San Jiao Finger Point. We inhale up from that point to the San Jiao Wrist Point, the San Jiao Elbow Point, and the San Jiao Shoulder Point, up to Baihui, and then we exhale the energy down to the Lower Dantian, which represents San Jiao for the purposes of this meditation.

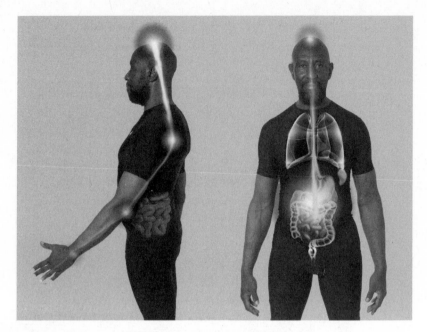

Figure 6.23: San Jiao Meridian

San Jiao Meridian	Location	Traditional Name
1. San Jiao Finger Point	Ulnar side of fourth finger nailbed	TH 1, Guanchong
2. San Jiao Wrist Point	Wrist depression on San Jiao line	TH 4, Yangchi
3. San Jiao Elbow Point	Flex elbow ninety degrees. Depression behind elbow tip.	TH 10, Tianjing
4. San Jiao Shoulder Point	Depression under the outermost part of the spine of shoulder blade	TH 14, Jianliao
5. Baihui	Crown	GV 20
6. San Jiao (Lower Dantian)	Fascia covering all the Organs, represented by the Lower Dantian	CV4, Guanyuan

Exercise 40: Empower the San Jiao Meridians

Part 1: Awaken the San Jiao Finger Point

1. Become aware of the right San Jiao Finger Point.

2. Form a Pearl at the right San Jiao Finger Point.

3. Chant the San Jiao Family Sound, Si. Feel the San Jiao Family and the point resonate as you chant. Integrate the point into the San Jiao Family. Repeat three times or more.

4. Repeat part 1 on the left side.

Part 2: Awaken the Rest of the
San Jiao Energy Points

5. Repeat part 1 with the San Jiao Wrist Points.

6. Repeat part 1 with the San Jiao Elbow Points.

7. Repeat part 1 with the San Jiao Shoulder Points.

8. Repeat part 1 at the Lower Dantian.

Part 3: Circulate the San Jiao Meridian Pearl

9. Become aware of your right San Jiao Finger Point. Inhale
    and form a Pearl at the right San Jiao Finger Point, and
    exhale the Pearl to the right San Jiao Wrist Point. Cycle
    the Pearl back and forth until that section of the Meridian
    becomes palpable.

10. Inhale the Pearl at the right San Jiao Wrist Point, and
    exhale it to the right San Jiao Elbow Point and back. Cycle
    the Pearl back and forth until that section of the Meridian
    becomes palpable.

11. Inhale the Pearl at the right San Jiao Elbow Point, and exhale
    it to the right San Jiao Shoulder Point and back. Cycle
    the Pearl back and forth until that section of the Meridian
    becomes palpable.

12. Inhale the Pearl at the right San Jiao Shoulder Point, exhale
    to Baihui, and inhale it back. Cycle the Pearl back and forth
    until that section of the Meridian becomes palpable.

13. Inhale the Pearl at Baihui, and exhale Baihui Qi to the San
    Jiao. Cycle the energy back and forth until that section of
    the Meridian becomes palpable.

14. Repeat part 3 on the left side.

Part 4: Empower the San Jiao Meridians

15. Become aware of the right San Jiao Finger Point and form a Pearl. Inhale the Pearl along the right San Jiao Meridian to Baihui.

16. As you exhale, chant Si, *sheeee* . . . Feel the vibration travel from Baihui to the the Lower Dantian. Repeat three times or more.

17. Abide in your Lower Dantian. Feel the quality of benevolence in your San Jiao. Awaken and bless your San Jiao.

18. Repeat part 4 on the left side.

Part 5: Integrate the Two Meridians

19. Inhale two Pearls from both San Jiao Finger Points along the San Jiao Meridians to Baihui. Chant Ha, *haaaaa* . . . as you direct the Pearl to the Lower Dantian. Feel the quality of benevolence in your San Jiao. Repeat three or more times.

20. Nourish your Qi. *I am in Qi; Qi is in me.*

The Gallbladder Meridian

The Gallbladder Meridian begins at the Gallbladder. A Gallbladder Qi Pearl is inhaled up to Baihui and exhaled down to the Navel, the Gallbladder Hip Point, the Gallbladder Knee Point, the Gallbladder Ankle Point, and finally to the Gallbladder Toe Point.

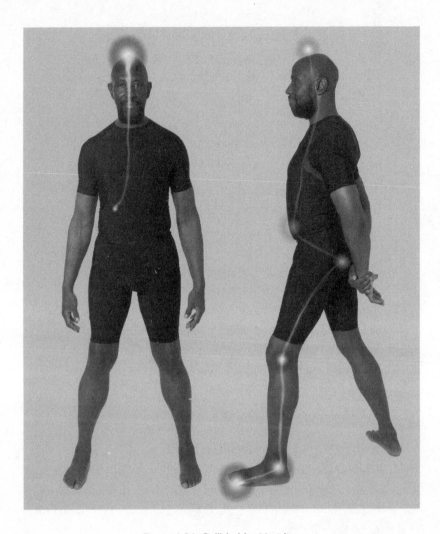

Figure 6.24: Gallbladder Meridian

Gallbladder Meridian	Location	Traditional Name
1. Gallbladder	Beneath liver on right side	
2. Baihui	Crown	GV 20
3. Navel	Belly button	CV 8
4. Gallbladder Hip Point	Sensitive point, 1/3 of the way from top of tailbone to hip bone	GB 30, Huantiao
5. Gallbladder Knee Point	In a depression below and in front of outer leg bone	GB 34, Yanglingquan
6. Gallbladder Ankle Point	In front and right below outer ankle point	GB 40, Qiuxu
7. Gallbladder Toe Point	Lateral side of fourth toe nailbed	GB 44, Zuxiaoyin

Exercise 41: Empower the Gallbladder Meridians

Part 1: Awaken the Navel

1. Become aware of the Navel.

2. Form a Pearl at the Navel.

3. Chant the Spleen Family Sound, Hu. Feel the Spleen Family and the point resonate as you chant. Integrate the point into the Spleen Family. Repeat three times or more.

Part 2: Awaken the Rest of the Gallbladder Energy Points

4. Repeat part 1 with the Gallbladder Hip Points.

5. Repeat part 1 with the Gallbladder Knee Points.

6. Repeat part 1 with the Gallbladder Ankle Points.

7. Repeat part 1 with the Gallbladder Toe Points.

8. Repeat part 1 with the Gallbladder.

Part 3: Circulate the Gallbladder Meridian Pearl

9. Become aware of your Gallbladder. Inhale Gallbladder Qi to Baihui and form a Pearl at the top of your head.

10. Exhale the Pearl to the Navel, and inhale it back to Baihui. Cycle the Pearl back and forth until that section of the Meridian becomes palpable.

11. Exhale the Pearl from the Navel to the right Gallbladder Hip Point, and inhale it back. Cycle the Pearl back and forth until that section of the Meridian becomes palpable.

12. Exhale the Pearl from the right Gallbladder Hip Point to the right Gallbladder Knee Point, and inhale it back. Cycle the Pearl back and forth until the pathway becomes clear and awareness of that section of the Meridian becomes palpable.

13. Exhale the Pearl from the right Gallbladder Knee Point to the right Gallbladder Ankle Point, and inhale it back. Cycle the energy back and forth until that section of the Meridian becomes palpable.

14. Exhale the Pearl from the right Gallbladder Ankle Point to the right Gallbladder Toe Point, and inhale it back. Cycle the energy back and forth until that section of the Meridian becomes palpable.

15. Repeat part 3 on the left side.

Part 4: Empower the Gallbladder Meridians

16. Become aware of the Gallbladder. Inhale a Gallbladder Qi Pearl to Baihui.

17. Form a Pearl at Baihui.

18. As you exhale, chant Hu, *whoooo* . . . Feel the vibration travel from Baihui along the right Gallbladder Meridian to the right Gallbladder Toe Point. Repeat three times or more.

19. Abide in the Qi flow of your Gallbladder Meridian. Feel the quality of benevolence flowing through your Gallbladder Meridian. Awaken and bless your Gallbladder Meridian.

20. Repeat part 4 on the left side.

Part 5: Integrate the Two Meridians

21. Inhale a Gallbladder Qi Pearl to Baihui, chant Hu, *whoooo* . . . and circulate two Pearls at the same time from Baihui along both Gallbladder Meridians to the Gallbladder Toe Points. Feel the quality of benevolence flowing though both Gallbladder Meridians. Repeat three or more times.

22. Nourish your Qi. *I am in Qi; Qi is in me.*

The Liver Meridian

The Liver Meridian begins at the Liver Toe Point. We inhale up from that point to the Liver Ankle Point, the Liver Knee Point, the Liver Thigh Point, the Navel, up to Baihui, and then we exhale the energy down to the center of the Liver.

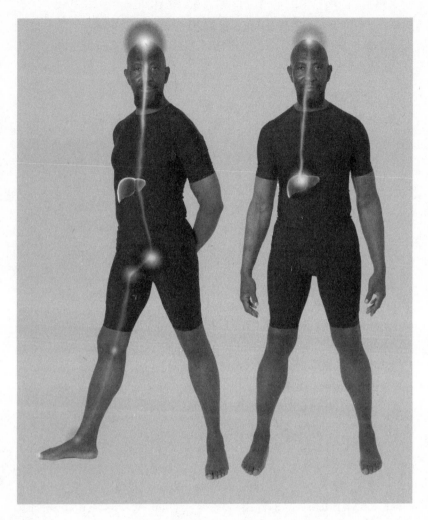

Figure 6.25: Liver Meridian

Liver Meridian	Location	Traditional Name
1. Liver Toe Point	Lateral side of first toe	LV 1, Dadun
2. Liver Ankle Point	Sensitive point in depression between the tendon and the inner ankle bone	LV 4, Zhongfeng
3. Liver Knee Point	Inner edge of knee crease when bent ninety degrees between the two hamstring tendons	LV 8, Ququan
4. Liver Thigh Point	Sensitive point on upper inner thigh about three inches below pubic bone	LV 10, Zuwuli
5. Huiyin	Perineum, midway between anus and genitals	CV 1
6. Baihui	Crown	GV 20
7. Liver	Below diaphragm, posterior to liver and spleen	

Exercise 42: Empower the Liver Meridians

Part 1: Awaken the Liver Toe Point

1. Become aware of the right Liver Toe Point.

2. Form a Pearl at the right Liver Toe Point.

3. Chant the Liver Family Sound, Xu. Feel the Liver Family and the point resonate as you chant. Integrate the point into the Liver Family. Repeat three times or more.

4. Repeat part 1 on the left side.

Part 2: Awaken the Rest of the Liver Energy Points

5. Repeat part 1 with the Liver Ankle Points.

6. Repeat part 1 with the Liver Knee Points.

7. Repeat part 1 with the Liver Thigh Points.

8. Repeat part 1 with Huiyin.

9. Repeat part 1 with the Liver.

Part 3: Circulate the Liver Meridian Pearl

10. Become aware of your right Liver Toe Point. Inhale and form a Pearl at the right Liver Toe Point, and exhale the Pearl to the right Liver Ankle Point. Cycle the Pearl back and forth until that section of the Meridian becomes palpable.

11. Inhale the Pearl at the right Liver Ankle Point, and exhale it to the right Liver Knee Point and back. Cycle the Pearl back and forth until that section of the Meridian becomes palpable.

12. Inhale the Pearl at the right Liver Knee Point, and exhale it to the right Liver Thigh Point and back. Cycle the Pearl back and forth until that section of the Meridian becomes palpable.

13. Inhale the Pearl at the right Liver Thigh Point, and exhale it to Huiyin and back. Cycle the Pearl back and forth until that section of the Meridian becomes palpable.

14. Inhale the Pearl at Huiyin, and exhale it to Baihui, and inhale it back. Cycle the Pearl back and forth until that section of the Meridian becomes palpable.

15. Inhale the Pearl at Baihui, and exhale Baihui Qi to the center of the Liver. Cycle the energy back and forth until that section of the Meridian becomes palpable.

16. Repeat part 3 on the left side.

Part 4: Empower the Liver Meridians

17. Become aware of the right Liver Toe Point and form a Pearl. Inhale the Pearl along the right Liver Meridian to Baihui.

18. As you exhale, chant Xu, *shewww* . . . Feel the vibration travel from Baihui to the Liver. Repeat three times or more.

19. Abide in your Liver. Feel the quality of benevolence in your Liver. Awaken and bless your Liver.

20. Repeat part 4 on the left side.

Part 5: Integrate the Two Meridians

21. Inhale two Pearls from both Liver Toe Points up the Liver Meridians to Baihui. Chant Xu, *shewww* . . . as you direct the Pearl to the center of the Liver. Feel the quality of benevolence in your Liver. Repeat three or more times.

22. Nourish your Qi. *I am in Qi; Qi is in me.*

Twelve Meridian Empowerment

Every twenty-four hours our Qi cycles around the Meridian Clock. Ideally, our day harmonizes with that rhythm, but realistically, for someone leading a modern lifestyle, that is unlikely. Eating patterns are disrupted. Sleeping patterns are disrupted. Life is complicated and it isn't always possible to adhere to the rhythm of the Qi Clock. The Twelve Meridian Empowerment combines the exercises we have been practicing into an integrated meditation practice. This meditation replicates the Qi flow of the Meridian Clock.

We begin by circulating a Sacred Pearl along the Lung Meridian, and this Pearl follows the Meridians in the order of the Meridian Clock until we end the cycle with the Liver Meridian. While we may not be able to line up our daily activities with the idealized timeframe, we can practice the Twelve Meridian Empowerment and align our energy body with the natural flow of an idealized lifestyle. My master, Xiao Yao, used to say that practicing one cycle of the Twelve Meridian Empowerment is equivalent to experiencing one daily cycle of the Meridian Clock. We can make up for deficiencies in our daily Qi flow by practicing this meditation.

And as we circulate the Sacred Pearl throughout the Meridian network, we spread Baihui Qi to all the Organs and the entire body. The Twelve Meridian Empowerment infuses the Organ Virtues with Baihui Qi. It endows goodwill with benevolence. It aligns Pure Mind and Higher Mind. There are two versions to the Empowerment. One version includes chanting, and the other version is practiced silently.

Exercise 43: Twelve Meridian Empowerment Meditation (Chanting Version)

Part 1: Opening

1. Adopt Natural Sitting Posture and practice Taiji Breathing for three cycles or more until your mind is calm.

2. Awaken Baihui and feel a divine presence hovering above you. Feel the energy of sacredness crowning your head.

Part 2: Meridian Chanting

3. Inhale a Lung Qi Pearl to Baihui at the top of your head. Feel the Pearl infuse with the quality of sacredness. As you exhale, chant the Lung Family Sound, Si, *szzzzz* . . . allow the Pearl to divide and circulate the two Pearls along both right and left Lung Meridians to the Lung Finger Points.

4. As you inhale, feel two Pearls form at the right and left Large Intestine Finger Points, and circulate the energy along the right and left Large Intestine Meridian lines to Baihui. Fuse the two Pearls at Baihui and exhale the energy from Baihui to anus at the end of the Large Intestine as you chant the Lung Family Sound, *szzzzz* . . .

5. Inhale a Stomach Qi Pearl to Baihui. Feel the Pearl infuse with the quality of sacredness. As you exhale, chant the Spleen Family Sound, Hu, *whoooo* . . . allow the Pearl to divide and circulate a Pearl along both right and left Stomach Meridians all the way down to the Stomach Toe Points.

6. As you inhale, feel two Pearls form at the right and left Spleen Toe Points, and circulate the energy along the right and left Spleen Meridian lines to Baihui. Fuse the two Pearls at Baihui, and exhale the energy from Baihui to the center of the Spleen as you chant the Spleen Family Sound, *whoooo* . . .

7. Inhale a Heart Qi Pearl to Baihui. Feel the Pearl infuse with the quality of sacredness. As you exhale, chant the Heart Family Sound, Ha, *haaaaa* . . . allow the Pearl to divide and circulate a Pearl along both right and left Heart Meridians all the way down to the Heart Finger Points.

8. As you inhale, feel two Pearls form at the right and left Small Intestine Finger Points, and circulate the energy along the right and left Small Intestine Meridian lines to Baihui. Fuse the two Pearls at Baihui, and exhale the energy from Baihui to the Small Intestine as you chant the Heart Family Sound, *haaaaa* . . .

9. Inhale a Urinary Bladder Qi Pearl to Baihui. Feel the Pearl infuse with the quality of sacredness. As you exhale, chant the Kidney Family Sound, Chui, *chuwee* . . . allow the Pearl to divide and circulate a Pearl along both right and left Urinary Bladder Meridians all the way down to the Urinary Bladder Toe Points.

10. As you inhale, feel two Pearls form at the right and left
    Kidney Foot Points, and circulate the energy along the right
    and left Kidney Meridian lines to Baihui. Fuse the two Pearls
    at Baihui, and exhale the energy from Baihui to the Kidneys
    as you chant the Kidney Family Sound, *chuwee* . . .

11. Inhale a Pericardium Qi Pearl to Baihui. Feel the Pearl infuse
    with the quality of sacredness. As you exhale, chant the San
    Jiao Family Sound, Xi, *sheeee* . . . Allow the Pearl to divide
    and circulate a Pearl along both right and left Pericardium
    Meridians all the way down to the Pericardium Finger Points.

12. As you inhale, feel two Pearls form at the right and left San
    Jiao Finger Points, and circulate the energy along the right
    and left San Jiao Meridian lines to Baihui. Fuse the two
    Pearls at Baihui and the energy from Baihui to San Jiao as
    you chant the San Jiao Family Sound, *sheeee* . . .

13. Inhale a Gallbladder Qi Pearl from your Gallbladder to
    Baihui. Feel the Pearl infuse with the quality of sacredness.
    As you exhale, chant the Liver Family Sound, Xu,
    shewww . . . allow the Pearl to divide and circulate a Pearl
    along both right and left Gallbladder Meridians all the way
    down to the Gallbladder Toe Points.

14. As you inhale, feel two Pearls form at the right and left Liver
    Toe Points, and circulate the energy along the right and left
    Liver Meridian lines to Baihui. Fuse the two Pearls at Baihui,
    and exhale the energy from Baihui to the center of your
    Liver as you chant the Liver Family Sound, *shewww* . . .

Part 3: Closing

15. Nourish your Qi. *I am in Qi; Qi is in me.*

You may also practice the Twelve Meridian Empowerment silently.
The instructions are presented below.

Exercise 44: Twelve Meridian Empowerment Mediation (Silent Version)

Part 1: Opening

1. Adopt Natural Sitting Posture and practice Taiji Breathing for three cycles or more until your mind is calm.

2. Awaken Baihui and feel a divine presence hovering above you and the energy of sacredness crowning your head.

Part 2: Meridian flow

3. Inhale a Lung Qi Pearl to Baihui, and exhale along the Lung Meridian to the Lung Finger Points.

4. Inhale Qi Pearls from the Large Intestine Finger Points to Baihui, and exhale Qi to the anus at the end of the Large Intestine.

5. Inhale a Stomach Qi Pearl to Baihui, and exhale along the Stomach Meridian to the Stomach Toe Points.

6. Inhale Qi Pearls from the Spleen Toe Points to Baihui, and exhale Qi to the center of the Spleen.

7. Inhale a Heart Qi Pearl to Baihui, and exhale along the Heart Meridian to the Heart Finger Points.

8. Inhale Qi Pearls from the Small Intestine Finger Points to Baihui, and exhale Qi to the center of the Small Intestine.

9. Inhale a Urinary Bladder Qi Pearl to Baihui, and exhale along the Urinary Bladder Meridian to the Urinary Bladder Toe Points.

10. Inhale Qi Pearls from the Kidney Foot Points to Baihui, and exhale Qi to the center of each Kidney.

11. Inhale a Pericardium Qi Pearl to Baihui, and exhale along the Pericardium Meridian to the Pericardium Finger Points.

12. Inhale Qi Pearls from the San Jiao Finger Points to Baihui, and exhale Qi to the Lower Dantian, which represents San Jiao.

13. Inhale a Gallbladder Qi Pearl to Baihui, and exhale along the Gallbladder Meridian to the Gallbladder Toe Points.

14. Inhale Qi Pearls from the Liver Toe Points to Baihui, and exhale Qi to the center of the Liver.

Part 3: Closing

15. Nourish your Qi. *I am in Qi; Qi is in me.*

The Twelve Meridian Empowerment saturates your energy body with a deep sense of sacredness and purity. Purity of your bodymind is a prerequisite for awakening Spirit. When goodwill and benevolence guide your thoughts and actions, you are like a ripe fruit. Your presence is sweet and nourishing. Your life is filled with good thoughts and good deeds. You incline toward virtue. When you are secretly blessing strangers and praying for their well-being, you are ready to take the next step and awaken as Spirit.

7

Huo Lu Gong Spirit Cultivation

The Gateway to Spirit

The Way of Virtue leads from Higher Mind to Pure Mind to Spirit. At each stage of spiritual development, your mind becomes increasingly refined, your virtue evolves, and your capacity for goodness grows. The Six Healing Sounds awakened your Organ Virtues, refined your moral character, developed your capacity for goodwill, and cultivated your Higher Mind. The Twelve Meridian Empowerment saturated your Organs and the Meridian network with Baihui Qi, endowed the Organ Virtues with benevolence, and cultivated Pure Mind. At this stage of the journey your mind is integrated and pure. You are inclined toward goodwill and benevolence.

The next step in the spiritual journey involves awakening the aspect of the mind that we call Spirit. The word "Spirit" is used in different ways by different people. Our definition of Spirit is precise and grounded in direct experience. Spirit arises when the mind is unified, undivided, and whole. When Spirit arises in awareness, we don't feel good. We don't even feel great. We feel perfect. Picture white light passing through a prism and fanning into a rainbow of colors. The refraction represents the Oneness of Spirit separating into the various aspects of duality.

The Six Healing Sounds and the Twelve Meridian Empowerment represent two steps that lead the mind back closer to the attainment of a unified mind, toward Spirit. Awakened Pure Mind stands at the boundary between Oneness and duality. Huo Lu Gong Spirit Cultivation is the name of the meditation practice presented in this chapter. This meditation unbends duality into Oneness. Metaphorically, Huo Lu Gong is the prism that your divided self passes on the way back to unified Spirit.

Huo Lu Gong unifies the mind and awakens Spirit by activating an Energy Point known as the Wuji Point. This point is a gateway that mediates between duality and Oneness. When that gate is closed, we are stranded in duality. Even when duality is blissful, delightful, pleasant, and filled with positive experiences, it is subject to change. Peace, the permanent attainment of well-being, still eludes the dualistic mind. Only when we awaken the Wuji Point and enter the realm of unified Oneness do we realize perfect and unchanging goodness.

The Wuji Point is subtle and inconspicuous. We can meditate for years and reach high levels of bliss but remain oblivious to its presence. It is ensconced deep inside the body, and activating the point requires a special method. Huo Lu Gong awakens the Wuji Point, and as our mind unifies as Spirit, we experience Perfect Peace and attain psychological wholeness. Daoist sages call the abode of Spirit the Primordial Realm, or Wuji. All spiritual traditions describe a veil that separates the phenomenal realm of duality from a transcendent realm of formless unity. A realm governed by division, ignorance, and sin separated from a realm governed by unity, perfection, and peace. In Christianity, the realm of peace is known as Heaven. In Islam, it is Paradise. In Buddhism, Nirvana. In theosophy, the Causal Plane. And when the mind abides in this dimension of wholeness, it experiences Perfect Peace, Shalom, Salam, Shanti, Moksha, or Salvation.

The realm of perfection that we experience when we awaken as Spirit is identified cross-culturally by many exalted names and described by supernal imagery. The names used to reference this reality are spoken with the utmost reverence. Those who enter this realm consciously are permanently transformed by the experience. They are permanently transfigured. Once you awaken as Spirit, your view of the phenomenal world is irrevocably changed, and your formless perfection becomes your foremost identity.

As we practice Huo Lu Gong, we part the veil of duality and enter the Primordial Realm where we attain Perfect Peace. We enter Wuji by awakening the Wuji Point. The Wuji Point cannot be awakened by forming a standard Pearl like the ones we used to awaken the Meridian Points. We need to apply a different energetic process to awaken this point. This process involves several steps that are then combined to yield the desired result. When the right formulation of energetic flows is achieved, the Wuji Point opens, and we awaken as Spirit.

The first step in Huo Lu Gong involves building a Qi Cauldron.

Step 1 Overview: Building a Qi Cauldron

A cauldron is a big pot used to cook food. The cauldron is filled with water. There is a fire under the cauldron that generates heat. The water begins to steam, ingredients are poured inside the cauldron, and we stir the pot. If you've ever prepared soup on a stove, you are familiar with these steps. Huo Lu Gong, Fire Oven Practice, replicates this process energetically. The cooking is going to take place inside your body, and the first step of the meditation is to build a Qi Cauldron that fits into your belly.

The Cauldron we are going to create matches your waistline. Imagine sliding a pot with a rounded bottom in the area around your belly at its widest girth. This Cauldron does not have legs. The pot is held in place by the Three Supports—your Navel and your two Kidneys. These Three Supports form an equilateral triangle. The pot is going to slide into your abdomen and be held securely in place by the Navel and two Kidneys. The rim of the pot will extend a few inches above the supports. Before we create the Qi Cauldron, we need to create the Three Supports. Squeeze your Navel and your two Kidneys and release. Become aware of the Three Supports.

The rounded bottom of the Qi Cauldron reaches all the way down to the top of your pubic bone. Visualize a pot held in place by your Navel and Kidneys, with a rim that extends around two inches above your Navel and a rounded bottom that extends down to your pubic bone. The Qi Cauldron is a big pot. The rounded bottom is important because you will be stirring the Qi Water in the pot, and a round bottom allows for more efficient stirring than a flat bottom.

The Qi Cauldron is made of Universal Qi. Universal Qi is the energy that you experience when you practice Nourishing Qi. Close your eyes for a moment and Nourish your Qi. *I am in Qi; Qi is in me* . . . The energy that arises in awareness when you are wallowing in the Qi of the Universe is the substance that you will use to create the Qi Cauldron. We create the Qi Cauldron by drawing Universal Qi through our forehead as we inhale. As you exhale, shape that energy into a Qi Cauldron with a rounded bottom and lower it until the top of the Qi Cauldron is wedged against the Three Supports. The rim extends slightly higher, and the bottom reaches the pubic bone. With practice, the Qi Cauldron becomes more tangible.

After the Qi Cauldron is in place, we fill it with Qi Water. Qi Water is made up of the energy of the Three Dantians and Baihui. We create a Pearl at the Lower, Middle, and Upper Dantians and inhale those three Pearls to Baihui. We infuse the qualities of Vitality, Love, and Wisdom with the sacredness of Baihui and spiral that energy into the Qi Cauldron.

Huo Lu Gong involves creating many energy whirls that spin in place or are circulated up and down like whirlwinds. These spinning energy structures can whirl outside the body or inside the body. They can expand and contract. They can whirl faster and slower. These whirls are symbolized by the Taiji symbol. These whirling Taijis can circulate Qi up or down efficiently and with great force. Picture a whirlwind raising a column of dust up in the air. Turn that image upside down and picture a whirling Taiji spiraling the energy of Baihui and the Three Dantians down into the Qi Cauldron. As you whirl the energy down, you feel the energies whirling around the core of your body down into the Qi Cauldron.

As the Qi Water fills the Qi Cauldron, the Taiji keeps on whirling. We feel the blended energy of Baihui and the Three Dantians stirring inside the pot. We feel the qualities of the Qi Water stirring all the way to the bottom of the pot. Qi Water is whirling from the waistline to the pubic bone. Sacredness, Wisdom, Love, and Vitality are stirring slowly and deeply inside your abdominal cavity.

The final part of step 1 involves dismantling the Qi Cauldron. We begin by inhaling the whirling Qi Water inside the Qi Cauldron up to the Upper Dantian. The energy whirls up to the center of the head, and when we feel the Taiji spinning inside our head we chant the sound of the Upper Dantian, Ong, *ongggg* . . . As we chant, we feel the resonance vibrate the center of our head and visualize the spinning Taiji turning violet. Violet is the color associated with Wisdom, the quality of the Upper Dantian. We chant Ong nine times, and each time we chant, the Taiji spins faster and faster. Then the Taiji whirls back down to the Qi Cauldron. It whirls back down without any color.

We repeat this process and raise whirling Qi Water to the Middle Dantian where we chant Ahh, *ahhhhh* . . . the chant of the Middle Dantian, nine times. As we chant, we feel the resonance vibrate the center of our chest and visualize the Taiji turning green. Green is the color associated with Love, the quality of the Middle Dantian. We chant Ahh nine times, and each time we chant, the Taiji spins faster and faster. The Taiji whirls back down to the Qi Cauldron. It whirls back down without any color.

The whirling Taiji returns to the Qi Cauldron where it gathers the remaining Qi Water as we chant Hong, *honggg* . . . nine times. As we chant, we feel the resonance vibrate the center of our lower abdomen and visualize the Taiji turning red. Red is the color associated with Vitality, the quality of the Lower Dantian. We chant Hong nine times, and each time we chant, the Taiji spins faster and faster.

Lastly, we transform the empty Qi Cauldron and any remaining Qi Water into a Qi Puddle. We inhale and chant Mmm, *mmmmmm* . . . This is the Universal Chant. It is intoned with the lips closed and the front teeth touching slightly. When you make the sound, your lips should vibrate distinctively. The Universal Chant is a calming, healing sound that can substitute for any other chant. It is a very adaptable sound that can be directed to any part of the body. We direct the Universal Chant to pump the Qi Puddle to the two Kidneys. As you chant Mmm, feel the vibration direct the Qi Puddle to your Kidneys. Feel your Kidneys absorb that energy. Finally, Nourish your Qi.

The formal instructions for step 1 of Huo Lu Gong are listed below.

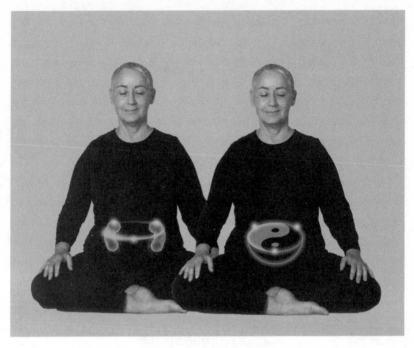

Figure 7.1: The Qi Cauldron

Exercise 45: Building a Qi Cauldron

Part 1: Creating the Three Supports

1. Adopt Natural Sitting Posture and practice Taiji Breathing for three cycles or more until your mind is calm.

2. Squeeze your Navel and release. Become aware of the Navel as a support.

3. Squeeze the two Kidneys and release. Become aware of the Kidneys as two supports.

4. Feel the Three Supports forming a stabilizing triangle to hold that Qi Cauldron in place.

Part 2: Creating the Qi Cauldron

5. Become aware of the Universal Qi outside your body. Inhale and absorb Universal Qi into your head through your forehead and shape it into a Qi Cauldron.

6. Exhale and direct the Qi Cauldron toward your belly.

7. Feel the Qi Cauldron settle securely in place on the Three Supports with the rim extending a few inches above the Navel. Feel the rounded bottom of the pot reaching down to your pubic bone.

Part 3: Creating Qi Water

8. Form a Pearl at the Lower Dantian in the center of your lower abdomen. Feel the concentration of Vitality Qi pulsating or spinning there.

9. Form a Pearl at the Middle Dantian in the center of your chest. Feel the concentration of Love Qi pulsating or spinning there.

10. Form a Pearl at the Upper Dantian in the center of your head. Feel the concentration of Wisdom Qi pulsating or spinning there.

11. Circulate all three Pearls up along the Central Meridian to Baihui. Begin with the Lower Dantian Pearl. Inhale it up to Baihui. Exhale. Inhale the Middle Dantian Pearl to Baihui. Exhale. Inhale the Upper Dantian Pearl to Baihui. Exhale.

12. Become aware of a Sacred Dantian Pearl forming at Baihui at the top of your head. Feel the Pearl begin to spin and expand into a Taiji. Allow the Pearl to spin around and around until it becomes a whirling Taiji.

13. Exhale and direct the whirling Taiji down toward the Qi Cauldron.

14. This whirling energy becomes the Qi Water that fills the Qi Cauldron. The Qi Cauldron is filled with a blend of whirling

Dantian Qi and Baihui Qi. Feel the essence of Wisdom, Love, and Vitality blended with the essence of sacredness whirling inside the Qi Cauldron.

15. Visualize a Taiji symbol spinning on the surface of the Qi Cauldron. Feel the Qi Water spinning slowly and deeply to the bottom of the pot. After some time, the whirling sensation continues effortlessly. Allow the Qi Water to spin for as long as you wish.

Part 4: Dismantling the Qi Cauldron

16. Inhale and whirl the Qi Water to your Upper Dantian at the center of your head. Exhale and chant Ong, the sound of the Upper Dantian, *ongggg* . . . Feel the Upper Dantian vibrate. As you chant Ong, feel the Taiji spin faster and faster and fill the Upper Dantian with the color violet. Chant Ong nine times. Then whirl the Taiji back to the Qi Cauldron.

17. Inhale and whirl the Qi Water to your Middle Dantian at the center of your chest. Exhale and chant Ahh, the sound of the Upper Dantian, *ahhhhh* . . . Feel the Middle Dantian vibrate. As you chant Ahh, feel the Taiji spin faster and faster and fill the Middle Dantian with the color green. Chant Ong nine times. Then whirl the Taiji back to the Qi Cauldron.

18. Inhale and whirl the remaining Qi Water in your Lower Dantian in your lower abdomen. Exhale and chant Hong, the sound of the Lower Dantian, *honggg* . . . Feel the Lower Dantian vibrate. As you chant Hong, feel the Taiji spin faster and faster and fill the Lower Dantian with the color red. Chant Ong nine times.

19. Inhale and transform the Qi Cauldron, the whirling Taiji, and any remaining Qi Water into a Qi Puddle. Exhale and chant the Universe Chant Mmm, *mmmmmm* . . . to pipe the

energy into both Kidneys. Feel the Kidneys absorb all the remaining energy.

20. Nourish your Qi. *I am in Qi, Qi is me.*

Step 2 Overview: Igniting the Qi Fire

Once you have a pot filled with water on a stove and you intend to make a soup, you need to start a fire. You turn the knob, and a spark is created that combines with the gas to ignite the fire. Qi Fire is created in a similar way. The gas that feeds Qi Fire is your sexual energy, and the knob that you turn to ignite the spark is produced by squeezing Huiyin, an Energy Point that we encountered previously. Huiyin means *Meeting of Yin*. It is located at the perineum, the midpoint between the anus and the genitals. Huiyin is located at the lower end of the Central Meridian and is diametrically opposed to Baihui, which is located at the upper end of the Central Meridian. Together, these two points define the central axis of the body.

While Baihui connects us to Heaven Qi, Huiyin connects us to Earth Qi. If you lose your balance and catch yourself before you fall, you have just activated Huiyin, your connection to the earth. Every time you take a step and feel your weight settle on the ground, you are pumping Earth Qi into Huiyin. Sitting in a deeply grounded squatting position such as Horse Stance also activates Huiyin. Huiyin is also associated with sexual energy. When we become sexually aroused, Huiyin becomes sensitized. Stimulating Huiyin when it is activated amplifies sexual desire, which is the goal of igniting Qi Fire.

To create Qi Fire, you inhale and hold your breath as you squeeze your anus and sexual Organs and release as you exhale. This action activates Huiyin. Squeezing and releasing is like turning the knob on a gas stove and creating the spark that will ignite the fire. We squeeze and release and feel a surge of sexual energy ignite the Qi Fire. To stabilize the Qi Fire, we direct a mild current of sexual energy to Huiyin. Without sexual energy, the Qi Fire is extinguished. With too much sexual energy, the sexual flame consumes us, and our meditation is disrupted. Our goal is to produce a low to moderate fire. We want Qi Water to be warm and comforting. Qi Water is never boiled.

As the warmth of the sexually charged Qi Fire rises from Huiyin, it warms the entire pelvic floor and extends up toward the rounded bottom of the Qi Cauldron, which is level with the pubic bone. As the warmth of the Qi Fire reaches the Qi Cauldron, the mild sexual charge of the Qi Fire is transmitted into the spinning Qi Water. As sexual energy and sacred energy mix, we experience a blissful feeling whirling inside our belly. The warm and mildly sexualized Qi Water is stirring slowly. The temperature is pleasant. The sensation is delightful and nurturing.

We control the intensity of the fire by squeezing and releasing the anus and sexual organs. That action is like pumping a bellows to make a fire bigger. Squeeze and release, squeeze and release, squeeze and release, and the mild Qi Fire becomes a moderate Qi Fire. As we increase the flow of sexual energy to Huiyin, the temperature of the Qi Water increases and the Taiji spins faster. The speed of the Taiji is moderated by the intensity of the sexual fire. We turn off the Qi Fire by switching off the flow of Huiyin Qi using our intention. This is like turning the knob into the off position on a stove.

In the following exercise, we ignite a Qi Fire at Huiyin and use that energy to warm the Qi Cauldron and the Qi Water. Then we turn the Qi Fire off.

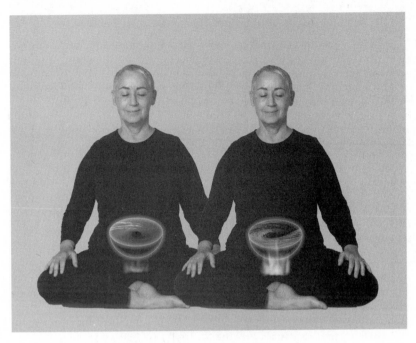

Figure 7.2: Igniting Qi Fire

Exercise 46: Igniting the Qi Fire

Part 1: Starting the Qi Fire

1. Adopt Natural Sitting Posture and practice Taiji Breathing for three cycles or more until your mind is calm.

2. Build a Qi Cauldron.

3. Become aware of Huiyin. (You can create a Pearl to awaken the Point.)

4. Squeeze and release your anus and genitals to create a spark of sexual energy at Huiyin.

5. Feel that spark ignite Huiyin Qi. Draw sexual energy from your genitals to Huiyin. Feel the Qi Fire intensify. Feel the warm Sexual Qi expand upward toward the rounded bottom of the Qi Cauldron. Feel the sensation of sexualized warmth spread into the Qi Water spinning inside the Qi Cauldron.

6. Squeeze and release your anus and genitals three times. Feel the mild Qi Fire grow into a moderate Qi Fire. Feel the extra warmth and sexual arousal energy warm the pelvic floor and extend upward toward the Qi Cauldron. Feel the sexual quality of Qi Fire blend with the sacred quality of Qi Water. Feel the elixir of Huiyin Qi, Baihui Qi, and Dantian Qi stirring inside the Qi Cauldron as the Taiji spins faster and faster.

7. Practice alternating between a mild fire and a moderate fire. Regulate the flow of your sexual energy by squeezing and releasing. Do not "boil" the Qi Water by adding too much sexual energy. If the sexual arousal becomes too strong, stop practicing and Nourish your Qi.

8. Continue stirring the mildly sexually charged Qi Water for as long as you wish.

Part 2: Turning Off the Qi Fire

9. Turn off the Qi Fire by shutting off the flow of sexual energy at Huiyin.

10. Dismantle the Qi Cauldron.

11. Nourish your Qi. *I am in Qi; Qi is in me.*

Step 3 Overview: Qi Steaming

Creating a Qi Cauldron, filling it with spinning Qi Water, and warming the Qi Water with Qi Fire are the prerequisites to creating Qi Steam. Qi Steaming is the key to awakening the Wuji Point and opening the gateway that leads to the Primordial Realm, Wuji. We create Qi Steam by controlling the spinning Taiji that is stirring the sexually charged Qi Water. As the Qi Fire becomes more intense, the Taiji spins faster and faster until a vortex forms at the center of the Taiji. As the Taiji spins, the root of that vortex extends downward. The vortex extends down half an inch below the surface. One inch. Two inches. As the Taiji spins, you feel your entire core whirling as the vortex draws your awareness down toward a focal point, the Wuji Point. The vortex of the spinning Taiji will be magnetically drawn to the Wuji Point. You will feel the tip of the vortex attracted toward this point, and once it reaches the right depth, it will lock in place and the Qi Steaming will begin.

The Wuji Point lies at the center of the Lower Dantian. Anatomically, the Wuji Point is located in front of the spine between the second and third lumbar vertebrae along the central axis that runs between Baihui and Huiyin. To find the physical location of the Wuji Point, place your second fingers on your left and right iliac crests, the most prominent aspect of your hips, and trace your fingers back toward your spine. Your fingertips will touch between the third and fourth lumbar vertebrae. Move up one vertebra and your fingers are level with the height of the Wuji Point. Project an imaginary line from your fingers on the spine toward the center of your body. Now picture the straight line connecting Baihui and Huiyin. The intersection between these two lines defines the location of the Wuji Point.

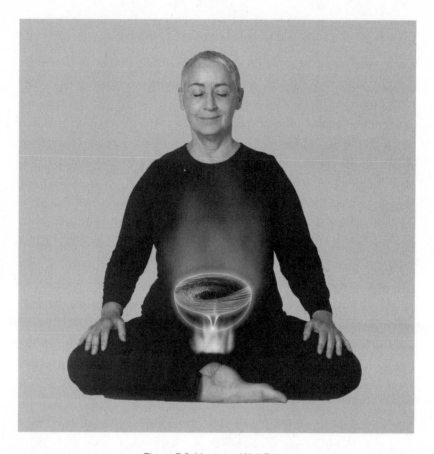

Figure 7.3: Vortex to Wuji Point

When the vortex of the spinning Qi Water reaches the Wuji Point, a fundamental energetic shift takes place and something magical happens. You feel as though a portal to another dimension opens up and a unique form of energy begins to flow into your body. Usually, when we circulate energy, we feel a current of Qi moving along a path through the physical body. We might even be able to project energy outside the body or absorb energy from another object like a tree or a flower into the body. Qi Steam is an altogether different experience. It is not an energy that we circulate in the conventional sense. As Qi Steam permeates the body, it feels like someone opened a valve and a mist pervades the body. We feel as though this mist is melting conventional reality and we are entering another world. Or perhaps, another world is entering us.

Imagine that you are in a steam room. Steam is passing through a valve and filling the room. At first the steam is thin, but over time it thickens until you can't see anything. This image helps us grasp the experience of Qi Steaming. As Qi Steam unfurls, it covers the body and extends beyond it. As Qi Steam spreads, our sense of boundaries dissolves and a wondrous spaciousness opens up. The feeling of our density as physical beings dissolves as well. As more Qi Steam is released, we experience ourselves as energetic beings. As we dissolve more fully into the spaciousness, our separate identity disappears, our thoughts disappear, our feelings disappear, and we become increasingly identified with the boundless spaciousness.

In Daoist mystical texts, Qi Steam is depicted as a cloud—the Primordial Cloud. Inside a cloud we can't see anything. Inside the Primordial Cloud, a boundless spaciousness opens up in all directions. Inside the Primordial Cloud, there is no inside and no outside. There are no distinctions to be made. There is no depth, there is no height. There is no up, there is no down. Just an endless expanse of formless space. There are no stray thoughts. No stray feelings. Just a peaceful stillness. Take away the impulses that form your sensations. Take away the desires that shape your thoughts and feelings. Take away the values that orient your attitudes and behaviors. Take away all the forms of consciousness, and what is left? Peace. Serenity. Perfection. Another name for the experience that arises when all desires are erased is Spirit.

The Primordial Realm dissolves the most basic categories we use to navigate Duality. Abiding as Spirit, we dissolve our sense of time and place. Meditation masters abiding as Spirit spend hours, days, weeks, months, and even years meditating in caves, requiring minimal food and water. Inside the Primordial Cloud, the hands of clock time dissolve. Inside the Primordial Cloud there is no distinction to be made between subject and object. There is no separate you and me. There is no us and them. These categories do not exist from the perspective of Spirit. Inside the Primordial Cloud there is no order, but everything is perfectly ordered. There is no structure, but everything is perfectly structured. No one is present, yet everyone is present. There is no sense of time, yet all time is here. There is no space, yet all space is here. There is no knowledge, yet all knowledge is here. Inside the Primordial Cloud, duality dissolves into Oneness.

A sense of deep well-being characterizes Oneness. The sensation is so deeply satisfying and soothing that our defenses dissolve. Our ego is extinguished. Psychological posturing drops away. Ambition evaporates. Fear vanishes. Inside the Primordial Cloud nothing changes because there are no pressing needs. There is no need to think because there are no problems to think about. Without needs and problems, dreams and wishes disappear. Without thoughts, suffering disappears. Without sensations, pain disappears. Without an identity, the ego disappears, and we emerge as boundless Spirit abiding in a boundless cloud of perfection. We become peace abiding in perfection.

Spirit is what remains of us once the manifold aspects of duality dissolve and we abide as Oneness. When our superficial and ephemeral identities are dissolved, we come to recognize our fundamental identity as Perfect Peace. Spirit is who we are when all differences and distractions are voided from perception. It is the answer to the question, *Who am I beyond the duality of life and death?* Spirit is your Original Self.

The quality of Perfect Peace that emanates from Spirit is known as Xian Tian Qi *(she-yan tee-yan)* or Primordial Qi. After we awaken Spirit and engage with the world saturated with Primordial Qi, we experience union with whatever we perceive. When we perceive the forest, we feel connected to every leaf on every tree. When we perceive the world, we feel connected to every human on every street. When we perceive ourselves, we feel intimately connected to the Dao. As Primordial Qi courses through our energy system, the One becomes the Many and the Many become the One. As we strengthen our connection to Spirit, our view of the world is spiritualized, and we come to realize the unity underlying all difference.

As Primordial Qi courses through the Meridian Network, the wholeness of our being becomes an emanation of peace. We experience the deepest sense of union with respect to ourselves and to everything else. Our personal relationships become imbued with the quality of peacefulness. We sense the spiritual interconnection of all things. Our presence inspires peace in the minds of others. We express our Organ Virtues in the service of peace. Kindness becomes kindness that pacifies. Courage becomes courage that encourages peace. The moral qualities of the Organs are spiritualized and are expressed in the pursuit of wholeness, union, and peace. As we cultivate Spirit through Huo Lu Gong, we develop a presence that inspires peace on earth.

When we are ready to end the Qi Steaming part of Huo Lu Gong, we create a gentle breeze with our breath to disperse the Primordial Cloud. The cloud precipitates into Qi Rain drops that fall into the Qi Cauldron. When the Primordial Cloud has dissipated, we end the meditation by turning off the Qi Fire and dismantling the Qi Cauldron. Qi Steaming may happen spontaneously the first time you try Huo Lu Gong, or it may take some time before the Wuji Point is activated. Allow the process to unfold naturally. With dedicated practice, you will eventually reach the goal.

Exercise 47: Qi Steaming

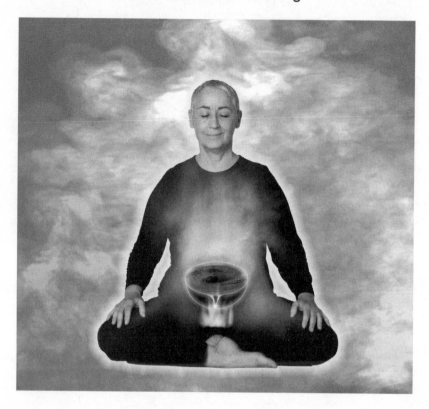

Figure 7.4: Qi Steaming

Part 1

1. Adopt Natural Sitting Posture and practice Taiji Breathing for three cycles or more until your mind is calm.

2. Create a Qi Cauldron.

3. Ignite the Qi Fire.

Part 2: The Primordial Cloud

4. Squeeze and release your anus and genitals to generate a moderate Qi Fire. Feel the Qi Fire warm the base of the Qi Cauldron. Allow the feeling of warmth to spread to the entire Qi cauldron and the Qi Water inside.

5. Feel the sexual energy of the Qi Fire blend with the sacred energy of Qi Water. As the Qi Water becomes warmer, the Taiji spins faster and faster.

6. Become aware of a vortex forming at the center of the Qi Cauldron on the surface of the spinning Qi Water. Squeeze and release. Squeeze and release. Feel the vortex extend deeper into the Qi Cauldron toward the Wuji Point.

7. Feel the root of the vortex become magnetized toward the Wuji Point. When the tip of the vortex connects with the Wuji Point, it will awaken. You will experience a distinctive sensation as the steaming process begins.

8. Feel Qi Steam misting internally. Allow the steam, Primordial Qi, to spread inside your body. Allow the natural intelligence of the Primordial Qi to follow its own path. As the Wuji Point continues to steam, the Primordial Cloud will grow thicker and thicker. Allow the Qi Steam to penetrate your Organs and tissues. Every cell of your body is warmed and soothed by Qi Steam.

9. Allow the mist to sink deeper into your body. Saturate your body with Primordial Qi. Your body feels nourished and cared for by this energy. Allow the steam to sink deeper into your body and mind. Your mind feels profoundly nourished and cared for by this energy. Allow your bodymind to settle into the stillness of Primordial Qi. Inside the Primordial Cloud you are at peace. Abide in Wuji. You are home. Abide in Perfect Peace.

Part 3: Qi Rain

10. Allow the Qi Steaming process to continue for as long as you wish. When the signal arises for you to end the meditation, it is time to disperse the Primordial Cloud.

11. Create a breeze with your breath. Inhale and exhale gently. Feel the Primordial Cloud dissipate into a mist of raindrops and direct that Qi Rain into the cauldron. When the Qi Rain stops and the cloud is dispersed, you are ready to end the practice.

Part 4

12. Dismantle the Qi Cauldron.

13. Nourish your Qi. *I am in Qi; Qi is in me.*

Step 4 Overview: Steaming the Organs

Daoist sages are often depicted as having childlike features and qualities. They are supple, like children. They smile like children. They are playful like children. They project an aura of childlike purity. The childlike imagery associated with Daoist adepts symbolizes the rejuvenation of the Organs and bodily tissues that occurs when we Qi Steam them. Primordial Qi is a regenerative energy, and when we direct it toward the Organs and their related body tissues, we restore in ourselves a quality of youthful exuberance.

As we steam the Organs, we also heal deep wounds held by the Organs and embedded throughout the body. These are the wounds that follow us day after day, for years, decades, and even across lifetimes. Qi steaming is like steam cleaning that helps us cleanse stubborn stains. Some wounds cannot be healed by the Six Healing Sounds or the Twelve Meridian Empowerment. These traumas remain trapped in the body and distort the mind. The deep sense of peace that we experience inside the Primordial Cloud enables the mind to drop all defenses. Our most vulnerable wounds are healed in the presence of Spirit. Primordial Qi can dissolve the imprint of our karmic wounds as it regenerates the Organs.

Picture a new laptop that runs perfectly well. It is in pristine condition the day you buy it. Five years later, it is malfunctioning. Viruses and malware are slowing it down. One of the keyboard keys is jammed and the metal casing is frayed. You send it in for repair. The techs replace the jammed key and polish the metal casing. They reset the software to factory settings and send you back what looks and feels like a brand-new computer. Imagine that you could send your Organs and tissues to a factory and get them reset. In fact, you can send your worn and torn bodymind in for a factory reset. That is what happens when you direct Qi Steam to the Organs and their related tissues. In the next series of exercises, we will steam the Organ Families with an expanded version and restore the body to its original luster.

Organ Steaming involves gathering an expanded set of qualities associated with each Organ Family. The extended members of the Organ Families that we collect include the Time of Day, Season, Taste, Noise, Weather, Body Fluid, Tissue, Expression, and Color. The blend of these qualities will be used to "flavor" the Qi Water that will be steamed. Until now, we have been steaming "plain" Qi Water, but when we Qi Steam the Organs, we introduce the blend of qualities associated with each Organ Family into the Qi Cauldron. Imagine throwing a blend of spices and herbs into boiling water and the fragrance of the steam filling the room. A blend of Italian spices and herbs is going to smell differently than Chinese spices and herbs. Similarly, the qualities of Liver Family Steam will be different than Kidney Family Steam.

Blending a dozen individual qualities associated with each Organ Family can become confusing and distracting, so to simplify that task, we distill those qualities into six vignettes. Each vignette is a scenario that captures the essence of a specific Organ Family. For example, the vignette of the Liver Family is a Warrior General waking up at sunrise and Shouting, *Good Morning!* That image captures the Essential Blend of the Liver Family. Distilling the twelve qualities associated with the Liver Family into that image makes it easy for us to grasp something that would otherwise be complicated.

The Essential Blend evoked by the vignette is drawn into a Taiji that is swirling around us like a whirlwind. We inhale the Taiji, through the sense organ associated with the Organ Family, into our head, and direct the whirling Taiji to Baihui at the top of our head. To continue with the Liver Family example, the qualities evoked by the image of the Warrior General are inhaled into the head through the Eyes and whirled up to Baihui. As we exhale, we direct the whirling Taiji infused with the Essential Blend into the Qi Cauldron and begin the Qi Steaming Process. During the steaming process, Primordial Qi and the fragrance of the Essential Blend seeps into every cell of the body. Finally, we disperse the Primordial Cloud into Qi Rain.

In the second part of Organ Steaming, we become aware of each member of the Organ Family whose Essential Blend we just steamed. For instance, if we are Steaming the Liver Family, we become aware of the Eyes. We inhale and whirl a Green Taiji (Green is the color of the Liver Family) from the Qi Cauldron to Baihui. The Green Taiji, which is infused with Primordial Qi, is blessed at the top of our head, and then we exhale, chant Xu, and direct the whirling Taiji to our Eyes. The spiritual blessing of Primordial Qi and Baihui Qi regenerates our Eyes. We repeat this process until every member of the Liver Family receives a spiritual blessing. Through this process, we restore our factory settings and our bodymind regenerates.

We repeat this process with all the Organ Families, and when we complete the Organ Steaming process, we dismantle the Qi Cauldron and end the meditation. The sequence of Organ Steaming follows the sequence of the Six Healing Sounds. We begin by Qi Steaming the Liver Family.

Qi Steaming the Liver Family

Liver Family Vignette: *The Warrior General wakes up at dawn and Shouts!*
The table below lists the extended members of the Liver Family.

Members of the Liver Family	
Archetype	Warrior General
Emotion	Enthusiastic Encouragement
Time of Day	Sunrise
Season	Spring
Taste	Sour
Noise	Shouting
Weather	Windy
Sense Organ	Eyes
Body Fluid	Tears
Tissue	Sinews
Expression	Nails
Color	Green

The Liver Family includes the Liver and the Gallbladder, which are associated with the archetype of the Warrior General. This combination is enthusiastic and courageous. It inspires hope and optimism. The new qualities associated with the Liver Family include East, Springtime, Green, Wind, Sour, and Shouting.

The eastern direction as an abstract concept does not invoke a quality, but when we realize that the sun rises in the East, we can attribute a meaningful quality to the direction. When we wake up in the morning, figuratively we are facing East. The day lies ahead full of potential, and our energy level is at its highest. The burst of energy that accompanies a night of wholesome sleep fills us with a sense of Enthusiasm and Encouragement. The feeling of dawn coincides with the feeling of East.

Spring invokes a similar feeling as dawn with respect to the seasons. In Spring, a new year full of possibilities dawns. The color Green is sprouting throughout the land. The Wind picks up. Sour is the taste that triggers alacrity. Bite into a lemon and you will experience the quality of dawn: Sour is analogous to morning and springtime at the level of taste. And Shouting plays a similar role at the level of locution. If someone Shouts at us, they invoke the quality of morning as we wake up and take notice.

To enhance our understanding of Liver Qi, we draw on the image of the Warrior General waking up on a bright Spring morning. He is full of vigor and pep. His nails are strong as claws. He has taut ligaments and tendons. The sun is rising over the Eastern horizon. It is Windy and his Eyes are tearing. The land is turning Green. He bites into a lemon and roars, "Good morning, I am awake!"

The image of the Warrior General waking up at dawn and Shouting captures the essence of Liver Family Qi.

Exercise 48: Steaming the Liver Family

Part 1: Taiji Outside Your Body

1. Adopt Natural Sitting Posture and practice Taiji Breathing for three cycles or more until your mind is calm.

2. Create a Qi Cauldron.

3. Ignite a mild Qi Fire.

4. Become aware of the space outside your body.

5. Invoke the energy of the Liver Family scenario: *The Warrior General wakes up at dawn and Shouts!* Invoke the qualities of Enthusiastic Encouragement, Sunrise, Spring, Sour, Tears, Sinews, and Green. Draw the essence of Liver Family Qi into a large Green Taiji spinning around you like a gentle whirlwind.

6. Inhale and draw the Green Taiji into your head through your Eyes. A Green Taiji is now spinning inside your head. Inhale and draw the Taiji to the top of your head. Exhale and chant Xu, *shewww . . .* as you direct the Green Taiji into the Qi Cauldron.

7. Feel the essence of the Liver Family Qi swirling inside the Qi Cauldron.

8. Begin steaming the Qi Water.

9. Abide in the Primordial Cloud. When you are ready, disperse the cloud into Qi Rain.

Part 2: The Spiritual Blessings

10. Become aware of the Green Taiji spinning in the Qi Cauldron.

11. Become aware of your Eyes. Inhale the Green Taiji to Baihui. Feel Primordial Qi and Baihui Qi blend. Exhale, chant Xu, *shewww . . .* and direct the spiritual blessing to your Eyes. Your Eyes are rejuvenated and healed.

12. Become aware of your Tears. Inhale the Green Taiji to Baihui. Feel Primordial Qi and Baihui Qi blend. Exhale, chant Xu, *shewww . . .* and direct the spiritual blessing to your Tears. Your Tears are rejuvenated and healed.

13. Become aware of your Ligaments and Tendons. Inhale the Green Taiji to Baihui. Feel Primordial Qi and Baihui Qi blend. Exhale, chant Xu, *shewww . . .* and direct the spiritual

blessing to your Ligaments and Tendons. Your Ligaments and Tendons are rejuvenated and healed.

14. Become aware of the Nails on your hands and feet. Inhale the Green Taiji to Baihui. Feel Primordial Qi and Baihui Qi blend. Exhale, chant Xu, *shewww* . . . and direct the spiritual blessing to your Nails. Your Nails are rejuvenated and healed.

15. Become aware of your Liver. Inhale the Green Taiji to Baihui. Feel Primordial Qi and Baihui Qi blend. Exhale, chant Xu, *shewww* . . . and direct the spiritual blessing to your Liver. Your Liver is rejuvenated and healed.

16. Become aware of your Gallbladder. Inhale the Green Taiji to Baihui. Feel Primordial Qi and Baihui Qi blend. Exhale, chant Xu, *shewww* . . . and direct the spiritual blessing to your Gallbladder. Your Gallbladder is rejuvenated and healed.

17. Become aware of your Liver Family. Inhale the Green Taiji to Baihui. Feel Primordial Qi and Baihui Qi blend. Exhale, chant Xu, *shewww* . . . and direct the spiritual blessing to your Liver Family. Your Liver Family is rejuvenated and healed.

Part 3: Closing

18. Dismantle the Qi Cauldron.

19. Nourish your Qi. *I am in Qi; Qi is in me.*

Qi Steaming the Heart Family

Heart Family Vignette: *The Emperor standing on the balcony at Noon is cheered on.*

The table below lists the extended members of the Heart Family.

Extended Members	Heart Family
Archetype	Discerning Emperor
Emotion	Refined Nobility
Time of Day	Noon
Season	Summer
Taste	Bitter
Noise	Laughing
Weather	Hot
Sense Organ	Tongue
Body Fluid	Sweat
Tissue	Blood Vessels
Expression	Complexion
Color	Red

The Heart Family includes the Heart and the Small Intestine, which are associated with the archetype of the Discerning Emperor, who is noble and judicious. This combination inspires admiration and joy. The new qualities associated with the Heart Family include South, Summer, Red, Heat, Bitter, and Laughter.

The southern direction corresponds to noontime, when the sun is at its highest peak and shines brightest. Noontime symbolizes charisma and nobility. Noontime is the imperial hour of the day. Summer is analogous to noontime at the level of the year. Light peaks at Noon in the summertime. The heat of Summer warms our Blood, which is Red, the color of the Heart. The Bitter taste helps to clear imbalanced heat from the Heart and helps us discern food that may be toxic and harmful. It helps the Tongue distinguish between foods that should be eaten from those that should be rejected.

Our vignette depicts the Emperor stepping onto his balcony at noon on a Summer day as his admirers cheer for him. This Emperor is not a dour-faced monarch, but a good natured bon vivant who brings joy to the people he loves.

The image of the Emperor waving warmly at the cheering crowd at Noon on a Summer day captures the essence of Heart Family Qi.

Exercise 49: Steaming the Heart Family

Part 1: Taiji Outside Your Body

1. Adopt Natural Sitting Posture and practice Taiji Breathing for three cycles or more until your mind is calm.

2. Create a Qi Cauldron.

3. Ignite a mild Qi Fire.

4. Become aware of the space outside your body.

5. Invoke the energy of the Heart Family scenario: *The Emperor standing on the balcony at Noon is cheered on.* Invoke the qualities of wholehearted joy, South, Summer, Red, Heat, Blood Vessels, Bitter, and Laughter. Draw the essence of Heart Family Qi into a large Red Taiji spinning around you like a gentle whirlwind.

6. Inhale and draw the Red Taiji into your head through your Tongue. A Red Taiji is now spinning inside your head. Inhale and draw the Taiji to the top of your head. Exhale and chant Ha, *haaaaa . . .* as you direct the Red Taiji into the Qi Cauldron.

7. Feel the essence of the Heart Family Qi swirling inside the Qi Cauldron.

8. Begin steaming the Qi Water.

9. Abide in the Primordial Cloud. When you are ready, disperse the cloud into Qi Rain.

Part 2: The Spiritual Blessings

10. Become aware of the Red Taiji in the Qi Cauldron.

11. Become aware of your Tongue. Inhale the Red Taiji to Baihui. Feel Primordial Qi and Baihui Qi blend. Exhale, chant Ha, *haaaaa* . . . and direct the spiritual blessing to your Tongue. Your Tongue is rejuvenated and healed.

12. Become aware of your Sweat. Inhale the Red Taiji to Baihui. Feel Primordial Qi and Baihui Qi blend. Exhale, chant Ha, *haaaaa* . . . and direct the spiritual blessing to your body temperature and Sweat. Your body temperature and Sweat are rejuvenated and healed.

13. Become aware of your Blood Vessels. Inhale the Red Taiji to Baihui. Feel Primordial Qi and Baihui Qi blend. Exhale, chant Ha, *haaaaa* . . . and direct the spiritual blessing to your Blood Vessels. Your Blood Vessels are rejuvenated and healed.

14. Become aware of your Complexion. Inhale the Red Taiji to Baihui. Feel Primordial Qi and Baihui Qi blend. Exhale, chant Ha, *haaaaa* . . . and direct the spiritual blessing to your Complexion. Your Complexion is rejuvenated and healed.

15. Become aware of your Heart. Inhale the Red Taiji to Baihui. Feel Primordial Qi and Baihui Qi blend. Exhale, chant Ha, *haaaaa* . . . and direct the spiritual blessing to your Heart. Your Heart is rejuvenated and healed.

16. Become aware of your Small Intestine. Inhale the Red Taiji to Baihui. Feel Primordial Qi and Baihui Qi blend. Exhale, chant Ha, *haaaaa* . . . and direct the spiritual blessing to your Small Intestine. Your Small Intestine is rejuvenated and healed.

17. Become aware of your Heart Family. Inhale the Red Taiji to Baihui. Feel Primordial Qi and Baihui Qi blend. Exhale, chant Ha, *haaaaa* . . . and direct the spiritual blessing to your Heart Family. Your Heart Family is rejuvenated and healed.

Part 3: Closing

18. Dismantle the Qi Cauldron.

19. Nourish your Qi. *I am in Qi; Qi is in me.*

Qi Steaming the Spleen Family

Spleen Family Vignette: *A playful stroll on a balmy Autumn Afternoon.*
The table below lists the extended members of the Spleen Family.

Extended Members	Spleen Family
Archetype	Charming Communicator
Emotion	Reassuring Clarity
Time of Day	Afternoon
Season	Indian Summer
Taste	Sweet

Noise	Singing
Weather	Damp
Sense Organ	Mouth and Lips
Body Fluid	Saliva
Tissue	Muscles and Flesh
Expression	Lips
Color	Yellow

The Spleen Family includes the Spleen and the Stomach, which are associated with the archetype of the Charming Communicator. This combination is clever and pleasant. It inspires wit and delight. The outer qualities associated with the Spleen Family include the Afternoon, Indian Summer, Yellow, Damp, Saliva, and Sweet.

If we wake up at 7:00 a.m. and go to bed around 10:00 p.m., the middle of the day takes place at 2:30 p.m. The pleasant energy of Afternoon resonates with the energy of the Spleen Family. In terms of the yearly cycle, Indian Summer, the pleasant window of time that takes place between late October and early November, when the leaves start turning Yellow, resonates with the Spleen and Stomach. The theme of pleasure, satisfaction, tantalizing dialogue, and movement resonate with Spleen Family Qi. Picture a couple on a first date on a balmy October afternoon. They are having a delightful conversation. They are flirting and enchanted by the witty dialogue. The tone of their voices is lyrical and if you heard them from a distance, you might think that they were Singing.

The image of a pleasant stroll on a balmy Autumn afternoon captures the essence of Spleen Family Qi.

Exercise 50: Steaming the Spleen Family

Part 1: Taiji Outside Your Body

1. Adopt Natural Sitting Posture and practice Taiji Breathing for three cycles or more until your mind is calm.

2. Create a Qi Cauldron.

3. Ignite a mild Qi Fire.

4. Become aware of the space outside your body.

5. Invoke the energy of the Spleen Family scenario: *A playful stroll on a balmy Autumn afternoon.* Invoke the qualities of Afternoon, Indian Summer, Yellow, Damp, Muscles and Flesh, Sweet, and Singing. Draw the essence of Spleen Family Qi into a large Yellow Taiji spinning around you like a gentle whirlwind.

6. Inhale and draw the Yellow Taiji into your head through your Mouth and Lips. A Yellow Taiji is now spinning inside your head. Inhale and draw the Taiji to the top of your head. Exhale and chant Hu, *whoooo . . .* as you direct the Yellow Taiji into the Qi Cauldron.

7. Feel the essence of the Spleen Family Qi swirling inside the Qi Cauldron.

8. Begin steaming the Qi Water.

9. Abide in the Primordial Cloud. When you are ready, disperse the cloud into Qi Rain.

Part 2: The Spiritual Blessings

10. Become aware of the Yellow Taiji in the Qi Cauldron.

11. Become aware of your Mouth and Lips. Inhale the Yellow Taiji to Baihui. Feel Primordial Qi and Baihui Qi blend.

Exhale, chant Hu, *whoooo* . . . and direct the spiritual blessing to your Mouth and Lips. Your Mouth and Lips are rejuvenated and healed.

12. Become aware of your Saliva. Inhale the Yellow Taiji to Baihui. Feel Primordial Qi and Baihui Qi blend. Exhale, chant Hu, *whoooo* . . . and direct the spiritual blessing to your Saliva. Your Saliva is rejuvenated and healed.

13. Become aware of your Muscles and Flesh. Inhale the Yellow Taiji to Baihui. Feel Primordial Qi and Baihui Qi blend. Exhale, chant Hu, *whoooo* . . . and direct the spiritual blessing to your Muscles and Flesh. Your Muscles and Flesh are rejuvenated and healed.

14. Become aware of your Lips. Inhale the Yellow Taiji to Baihui. Feel Primordial Qi and Baihui Qi blend. Exhale, chant Hu, *whoooo* . . . and direct the spiritual blessing to your Lips. Your Lips are rejuvenated and healed.

15. Become aware of your Spleen. Inhale the Yellow Taiji to Baihui. Feel Primordial Qi and Baihui Qi blend. Exhale, chant Hu, *whoooo* . . . and direct the spiritual blessing to your Spleen. Your Spleen is rejuvenated and healed.

16. Become aware of your Stomach. Inhale the Yellow Taiji to Baihui. Feel Primordial Qi and Baihui Qi blend. Exhale, chant Hu, *whoooo* . . . and direct the spiritual blessing to your Stomach. Your Stomach is rejuvenated and healed.

17. Become aware of your Spleen Family. Inhale the Yellow Taiji to Baihui. Feel Primordial Qi and Baihui Qi blend. Exhale, chant Hu, *whoooo* . . . and direct the spiritual blessing to your Spleen Family. Your Spleen Family is rejuvenated and healed.

Part 3: Closing

18. Dismantle the Qi Cauldron.

19. Nourish your Qi. *I am in Qi; Qi is in me.*

Qi Steaming the Lung Family

Lung Family Vignette: *Soulmates holding hands at Sunset.*
The table below lists the extended members of the Lung Family.

Extended Members	Lung Family
Archetype	Trusted Soulmate
Emotion	Honest Kindness
Time of Day	Sunset
Season	Late Autumn
Taste	Pungent
Noise	Crying
Weather	Dry
Sense Organ	Nose
Body Fluid	Mucus
Tissue	Skin
Expression	Body Hair
Color	White

The Lung Family includes the Lungs and the Large Intestine, which are associated with the archetype of the Trusted Soulmate. This combination is kind and honest. It inspires trust and intimacy. The outer qualities associated with the Lung Family include West, Sunset, White, Late Autumn, Dryness, Spiciness, and Crying.

The western direction corresponds to Sunset, when the sun dips over the western horizon. The day is about to end, and evening is about to begin. This moment exemplifies the turning tides between day and night. The season that corresponds to Sunset is late Autumn, when the tide of the year is turning. Leaves have fallen and the branches are bare. The year is about to end, and endings inspire sadness and nostalgia. In Chinese culture, the color White is associated with death and symbolizes sadness and loss. As the temperature makes a noticeable drop, we begin to feel the dry and penetrating chill. These qualities inspire an inward turn. Yin is waxing during this time. We become more introverted. We seek warmth and human contact. Spicy foods that raise our core temperature are also associated with Late Autumn.

The image of Soulmates holding hands at Sunset captures the essence of Lung Family Qi.

Exercise 51: Steaming the Lung Family

Part 1: Taiji outside your body

1. Adopt Natural Sitting Posture and practice Taiji Breathing for three cycles or more until your mind is calm.

2. Create a Qi Cauldron.

3. Ignite a mild Qi Fire.

4. Become aware of the space outside your body.

5. Invoke the energy of the Lung Family scenario: *Soulmates holding hands at Sunset.* Invoke the qualities of Sunset, Late Autumn, White, Dry, Skin, Body Hair, Pungent, and Crying. Draw the essence of Lung Family Qi into a large White Taiji spinning around you like a gentle whirlwind.

6. Inhale and draw the White Taiji into your head through your Nose. A White Taiji is now spinning inside your head. Inhale and draw the Taiji to the top of your head. Exhale and chant Si, *szzzzz* . . . as you direct the White Taiji into the Qi Cauldron.

7. Feel the essence of the Lung Family Qi swirling inside the Qi Cauldron.

8. Begin steaming the Qi Water.

9. Abide in the Primordial Cloud. When you are ready, disperse the cloud into Qi Rain.

Part 2: The Spiritual Blessings

10. Become aware of the White Taiji in the Qi Cauldron.

11. Become aware of your Nose. Inhale the White Taiji to Baihui. Feel Primordial Qi and Baihui Qi blend. Exhale, chant Si, *szzzzz* . . . and direct the spiritual blessing to your Nose. Your Nose is rejuvenated and healed.

12. Become aware of your Mucus. Inhale the White Taiji to Baihui. Feel Primordial Qi and Baihui Qi blend. Exhale, chant Si, *szzzzz* . . . and direct the spiritual blessing to your Mucus. Your Mucus is rejuvenated and healed.

13. Become aware of your Skin. Inhale the White Taiji to Baihui. Feel Primordial Qi and Baihui Qi blend. Exhale, chant Si, *szzzzz* . . . and direct the spiritual blessing to your Skin. Your Skin is rejuvenated and healed.

14. Become aware of your Body Hair. Inhale the White Taiji to Baihui. Feel Primordial Qi and Baihui Qi blend. Exhale, chant Si, *szzzzz* . . . and direct the spiritual blessing to your Body Hair. Your Body Hair is rejuvenated and healed.

15. Become aware of your Lungs. Inhale the White Taiji to Baihui. Feel Primordial Qi and Baihui Qi blend. Exhale, chant Si, *szzzzz* . . . and direct the spiritual blessing to your Lungs. Your Lungs are rejuvenated and healed.

16. Become aware of your Large Intestine. Inhale the White Taiji to Baihui. Feel Primordial Qi and Baihui Qi blend. Exhale, chant Si, *szzzzz* . . . and direct the spiritual blessing to your Large Intestine. Your Large Intestine is rejuvenated and healed.

17. Become aware of your Lung Family. Inhale the White Taiji to Baihui. Feel Primordial Qi and Baihui Qi blend. Exhale, chant Si, *szzzzz* . . . and direct the spiritual blessing to your Lung Family. Your Lung Family is rejuvenated and healed.

Part 3: Closing

18. Dismantle the Qi Cauldron.

19. Nourish your Qi. *I am in Qi; Qi is in me.*

Qi Steaming the Kidney Family

Kidney Family Vignette: *A Mystic meditating at Midnight in Winter.*

The table below lists the extended members of the Kidney Family.

Extended Members	Kidney Family
Archetype	Tough Old Bird
Emotion	Unbendable Willpower
Time of Day	Midnight
Season	Winter
Taste	Salty
Noise	Groaning
Weather	Cold
Sense Organ	Ears
Body Fluid	Bone Marrow
Tissue	Bones
Expression	Head Hair
Color	Ocean Blue

The Kidney Family includes the Kidneys and the Urinary Bladder, which are associated with the archetype of the Tough Old Bird. This combination is disciplined, resilient, and independent. It inspires persistence through adversity. The outer qualities associated with the Kidney Family include North, Midnight, Winter, Ocean Blue, Cold, Salty, and Groaning.

North corresponds to the position of the sun at Midnight when the sky is darkest. It is a time of silence and inwardness. It is a time of caution. Nature is invisible at night and the one place that we can retreat to at that time is the inner world of dreams and meditation. Winter is inhospitable and brutally cold. We encounter the harshness of the frigid air and Groan in response. Winter is brutal. We embody the archetype of the Tough Old Bird to overcome the adversity. Winter pressures us into becoming more resilient and disciplined. Without a steely will, we can't survive the challenge of Winter and Midnight. Both can be frightening in their own way, and both inspire caution. The color of the Kidneys is dark Ocean Blue. The taste associated with Winter is Salty, the taste of ocean water. Kidney time is associated with maximum Yin, when light is a distant memory, the doors to the imagination are open wide, and awareness withdraws most easily inwardly.

The image of a Mystic meditating at Midnight in Winter captures the essence of Kidney Family Qi.

Exercise 52: Steaming the Kidney Family

Part 1: Taiji Outside Your Body

1. Adopt Natural Sitting Posture and practice Taiji Breathing for three cycles or more until your mind is calm.

2. Create a Qi Cauldron.

3. Ignite a mild Qi Fire.

4. Become aware of the space outside your body.

5. Invoke the energy of the Kidney Family scenario: *A Mystic meditating at Midnight in Winter.* Invoke the qualities of Midnight, Winter, Ocean Blue, Cold, Bones, Bone Marrow, Salty, and Groaning. Draw the essence of Kidney Family Qi into a large Ocean Blue Taiji spinning around you like a gentle whirlwind.

6. Inhale and draw the Ocean Blue Taiji into your head through your Ears. A Ocean Blue Taiji is now spinning inside your head. Inhale and draw the Taiji to the top of your head. Exhale and chant Chui, *chuwee . . .* as you direct the Ocean Blue Taiji into the Qi Cauldron.

7. Feel the essence of the Kidney Family Qi swirling inside the Qi Cauldron.

8. Begin steaming the Qi Water.

9. Abide in the Primordial Cloud. When you are ready, disperse the cloud into Qi Rain.

Part 2: The Spiritual Blessings

10. Become aware of the Ocean Blue Taiji in the Qi Cauldron.

11. Become aware of your Ears. Inhale the Ocean Blue Taiji to Baihui. Feel Primordial Qi and Baihui Qi blend. Exhale, chant Chui, *chuwee* . . . and direct the spiritual blessing to your Ears. Your Ears are rejuvenated and healed.

12. Become aware of your Bone Marrow. Inhale the Ocean Blue Taiji to Baihui. Feel Primordial Qi and Baihui Qi blend. Exhale, chant Chui, *chuwee* . . . and direct the spiritual blessing to your Bone Marrow. Your Bone Marrow is rejuvenated and healed.

13. Become aware of your Bones. Inhale the Ocean Blue Taiji to Baihui. Feel Primordial Qi and Baihui Qi blend. Exhale, chant Chui, *chuwee* . . . and direct the spiritual blessing to your Bones. Your Bones are rejuvenated and healed.

14. Become aware of your Head Hair. Inhale the Ocean Blue Taiji to Baihui. Feel Primordial Qi and Baihui Qi blend. Exhale, chant Chui, *chuwee* . . . and direct the spiritual blessing to your Head Hair. Your Head Hair is rejuvenated and healed.

15. Become aware of your Kidneys. Inhale the Ocean Blue Taiji to Baihui. Feel Primordial Qi and Baihui Qi blend. Exhale, chant Chui, *chuwee* . . . and direct the spiritual blessing to your Kidneys. Your Kidneys are rejuvenated and healed.

16. Become aware of your Urinary Bladder. Inhale the Ocean Blue Taiji to Baihui. Feel Primordial Qi and Baihui Qi blend. Exhale, chant Chui, *chuwee* . . . and direct the spiritual blessing to your Urinary Bladder. Your Urinary Bladder is rejuvenated and healed.

17. Become aware of your Kidney Family. Inhale the Ocean Blue Taiji to Baihui. Feel Primordial Qi and Baihui Qi blend. Exhale, chant Chui, *chuwee* . . . and direct the spiritual blessing to your Kidney Family. Your Kidney Family is rejuvenated and healed.

Part 3: Closing

18. Dismantle the Qi Cauldron.

19. Nourish your Qi. *I am in Qi; Qi is in me.*

Qi Steaming the San Jiao Family

San Jiao Family Vignette: *A Mother holding an infant while humming a lullaby.*

The table below lists the extended members of the San Jiao Family.

Extended Members	San Jiao Family
Archetype	Compassionate Mother
Emotion	Warmhearted Unity
Time of Day	All Times
Season	All Seasons
Taste	All Flavors

Noise	Harmonious Sounds
Weather	All Weather
Sense Organ	Face
Body Fluid	Extracellular Fluids
Tissue	All Fascia
Expression	Overall Demeanor
Color	Violet

The San Jiao Family includes San Jiao and the Pericardium, which are associated with the archetype of the Compassionate Mother. This combination inspires harmony and a sense of unity. It inspires singleness of purpose and care. The outer qualities associated with the San Jiao Family include All Times of Day, All Seasons, All Weather, All Harmonious Flavors and Sounds, Fascia, Extracellular Fluids, and the color Violet. Imagine that you are at the center of the sun looking out at the entire solar system. There is no season and there is no time of day from that perspective. San Jiao embraces wholeness and all perspectives. When we embrace wholeness by standing at the center, we notice that everything is in relationship to everything else. From space, you can see day and night simultaneously on the surface of the earth. You can see winter and summer simultaneously. All perspectives are unified. The ability to unify and care for the whole captures the essence of the San Jiao Family.

The image of a Mother holding an infant while humming a lullaby captures the essence of San Jiao Family Qi.

Exercise 53: Steaming the San Jiao Family

Part 1: Taiji outside your body

1. Adopt Natural Sitting Posture and practice Taiji Breathing for three cycles or more until your mind is calm.

2. Create a Qi Cauldron.

3. Ignite a mild Qi Fire.

4. Become aware of the space outside your body.

5. Invoke the energy of the San Jiao Family scenario: *A Mother holding an infant while humming a lullaby.* Invoke all the qualities of All Times and Seasons, Violet, Cold, Fascia, Extracellular Fluids, and All Harmonious Flavors and Sounds. Draw the essence of San Jiao Family Qi into a large Violet Taiji spinning around you like a gentle whirlwind.

6. Inhale and draw the Violet Taiji into your head through your Face. A Violet Taiji is now spinning inside your head. Inhale and draw the Taiji to the top of your head. Exhale and chant Xi, *sheeee . . .* as you direct the Violet Taiji into the Qi Cauldron.

7. Feel the essence of the San Jiao Family Qi swirling inside the Qi Cauldron.

8. Begin steaming the Qi Water.

9. Abide in the Primordial Cloud. When you are ready, disperse the cloud into Qi Rain.

Part 2: The Spiritual Blessings

10. Become aware of the Violet Taiji in the Qi Cauldron.

11. Become aware of your Face. Inhale the Violet Taiji to Baihui. Feel Primordial Qi and Baihui Qi blend. Exhale, chant Xi, *sheeee . . .* and direct the spiritual blessing to your Face. Your Face is rejuvenated and healed.

12. Become aware of your Fascia. Inhale the Violet Taiji to Baihui. Feel Primordial Qi and Baihui Qi blend. Exhale, chant Xi, *sheeee* . . . and direct the spiritual blessing to your Fascia. Your Fascia is rejuvenated and healed.

13. Become aware of your Extracellular Fluids and lymphatic fluid. Inhale the Violet Taiji to Baihui. Feel Primordial Qi and Baihui Qi blend. Exhale, chant Xi, *sheeee* . . . and direct the spiritual blessing to your Extracellular Fluids. Your Extracellular Fluids are rejuvenated and healed.

14. Become aware of your Overall Expression, the way that you come off as a human being. Inhale the Violet Taiji to Baihui. Feel Primordial Qi and Baihui Qi blend. Exhale, chant Xi, *sheeee* . . . and direct the spiritual blessing to your Overall Expression. Your Overall Expression is rejuvenated and healed.

15. Become aware of San Jiao, the tissues that hold your body parts together. Inhale the Violet Taiji to Baihui. Feel Primordial Qi and Baihui Qi blend. Exhale, chant Xi, *sheeee* . . . and direct the spiritual blessing to San Jiao. Your San Jiao is rejuvenated and healed.

16. Become aware of your Pericardium. Inhale the Violet Taiji to Baihui. Feel Primordial Qi and Baihui Qi blend. Exhale, chant Xi, *sheeee* . . . and direct the spiritual blessing to your Pericardium. Your Pericardium is rejuvenated and healed.

17. Become aware of your San Jiao Family. Inhale the Violet Taiji to Baihui. Feel Primordial Qi and Baihui Qi blend. Exhale, chant Xi, *sheeee* . . . and direct the spiritual blessing to your San Jiao Family. Your San Jiao Family is rejuvenated and healed.

Part 3: Closing

18. Dismantle the Qi Cauldron.

19. Nourish your Qi. *I am in Qi; Qi is in me.*

The Heart, the Crown, Spirit, and Virtue

Your body is a temple filled with hidden treasures. Your Organ Families, the Meridians and their Points, the Wuji Point, your Dantians, the Central Meridian, Baihui, and Huiyin are some of the spiritual jewels that await your discovery. As you uncover these riches, the quality of your life improves. My master, Xiao Yao, was a poor man. He didn't own anything. And yet Xiao Yao was the wealthiest man I ever met. He reveled in the spiritual treasures that are hidden inside each one of us. The Way of Virtue is the most rewarding path a human being can pursue. Eventually, we all die. The temple that embodies us turns to dust. But our awareness continues the journey toward Dao adorned in the spiritual jewels that we unearthed over our lifetime.

As you develop proficiency with the Six Healing Sounds, the Twelve Meridian Empowerment, and Huo Lu Gong, you will become increasingly aware of the new energies you cultivated, forming positive feelings and thoughts. Your energy body will become adorned in spiritual jewels. You will aspire to blessing others, especially those who suffer and are unaware of their spiritual nature. You will emanate an aura of peace and your presence will transform confusion into creative order. As you embody the energies awakened by these practices, you will become a guiding light on the Way of Virtue and inspire others to discover and walk this path. In the name of whichever Supreme Ultimate that you may worship, in the name of the lineage that has blessed me with the knowledge that I share, in the name of my master Xiao Yao, may Dao bless you with a healthy and virtuous life.

Below are the instructions to the final exercise, Huo Lu Gong.

Exercise 54: Huo Lu Gong Spirit Cultivation

As you practice Huo Lu Gong, become aware of the benefic spiritual presence saturating your body. Become aware of the Wuji Point as the center of a sacred circle that blesses and empowers your being. Become aware of your goodness radiating as pure light. Realize that as you practice, you bless yourself and brighten creation. Most importantly, as you practice, revel in the peace.

Part 1

1. Create a Qi Cauldron.

2. Create a mild Qi Fire.

Part 2

3. Steam the Liver Family.

4. Steam the Heart Family.

5. Steam the Spleen Family.

6. Steam the Lung Family.

7. Steam the Kidney Family.

8. Steam the San Jiao Family.

Part 3

9. Dismantle the Qi Cauldron.

10. Nourish your Qi. *I am in Qi; Qi is in me.*

Opening the Door to Another World

Our journey began with a series of questions about the mystery of life, death, and existence. Daoist sages understood that meaningful answers to the biggest questions cannot be answered by mere words. Spiritual wisdom transcends grammar, reason, and the senses. These questions can only be understood experientially. Wisdom is revealed to us gradually as we awaken and embody our true nature. If you have followed along and cultivated your Spirit, by now you identify as spirit-in-the-world. You perceive the One and the Many as expressions of a seamless whole that is fluid and in constant relationship to its parts. You realize that the perennial questions are best answered by realizing your spiritual nature.

The practices described in The Way of Virtue represent the halfway mark on the journey to Dao. Once we awaken as spirit, our vision of the world is intimately transformed and we experience unimaginable degrees of peace, but even more wholistic and rarefied stages of development lie ahead. Spirit itself can be cultivated. Spirit can grow, mature, and unfold in subtle ways that reveal deeper truths about the mystery of existence. Consider identifying as the Pacific Ocean. The depth and breadth of the ocean is awesome and seemingly endless. This vision represents the stage of Huo Lu Gong. But now consider the Pacific Ocean from the vantage point of outer space. The earth is a tiny drop in an ocean of emptiness that extends out to the farthest reaches of our universe. We have opened a door to another world, yet beyond this wondrous new world lies another that is even more remarkable. As Xiao Yao used to say, beyond this sky lies another sky.

As spirit matures, boundaries soften, and our vision of reality becomes dreamlike. We identify with the dream-maker that forges the mind that shapes the world. Eventually, the boundary between the individual mind and the world dissolves into the stillness of the Supreme Ultimate void that permeates all that is. From a higher spiritual vantage point, we are sharing the dreams of ten thousand lifetimes in timeless, spaceless nonbeing. May the ever-present and all-encompassing Supreme Ultimate bless and guide your spirit toward Dao. May your spirit someday dissolve into the stillness of nonbeing. And in the meantime, I invite you into my dream . . .

Epilogue

A Dream, Imagined

I awaken in a golden meadow under a golden sky sitting cross-legged on lush grass. There are a handful of others, also seated, and we are all wearing silken white tunics and white pants. We are facing a windblown bristlecone pine. The braided bark twists upon itself and the branches point upward like gnarly wooden digits. A man is sitting cross-legged at the foot of the tree. The space around him exudes a peaceful aura punctuated by his penetrating gaze. His hands are resting on his lap in meditative repose. He has a prominent forehead, long white bushy brows, and receding white hair that drapes over his shoulders. A fine white beard reaches down to the center of his chest. He is draped in a white tunic bordered by a golden fringe. His pupils sparkle as he makes eye contact with me. Crystal clarity is radiating from his eyes and the serenity of his smile is unmistakable. I feel at ease in this welcoming space. I feel at home in the presence of this sage.

Far beyond this realm, yet intimately close, my physical body is asleep under a thick white comforter. The alarm clock on the night table reads 3:17 a.m. A gray owl lands on the branch of a tree in my yard and flutters away. The night sky is clear, and the planet Saturn is rising over the tree line as a silver crescent moon hovers overhead. The stars are shimmering as the blinking light of an airplane is cutting east across the heavens, readying for a transatlantic voyage. The passengers on the plane are mostly asleep, but one of them is awake and reflecting on the cryptic words his wife texted before takeoff.

"Good news," she wrote. "We'll talk when you're back home. Bon voyage."

At this same instant, it is morning in the European hamlet where this nameless traveler lives, and his wife is on a tram. She opens her purse and glances at the test strip to make sure it is still indicating positive. Boy or girl, she wonders, and smiles. An elderly man with a downcast expression holding a bouquet of wildflowers is seated next to her. He is on his way to the hospital to visit his wife. She is not faring well, and he ponders her fate. He gets off at the next stop. On the way to the hospital, he encounters an acquaintance from his university days. The two men exchange a few words, shake hands, and part ways.

The acquaintance is holding a brown paper bag filled with bread-crumbs. He walks toward a bench on the sidewalk and sits. He throws crumbs on the ground and cooing pigeons gather around him bobbing heads and pecking the ground. Now retired, he delights in feeding the birds. A young woman in a red jacket walks past the bobbing birds at a brisk pace. She crosses the street and walks down another on her way to work. As she walks by a bookstore that sells used books, she stops abruptly. She is in a hurry, but she feels curiously compelled to go inside. She peruses the aisles randomly. She picks a slim yellow jacket that catches her attention. It is *The Dao De Jing*. She flips the book open to the first chapter and reads.

> The Dao that can be named is not the absolute Dao. The name that can be spoken is not the name of the eternal. The unmanifest eternal Dao is the origin of Heaven and Earth. Manifest, it becomes the mother of all things. Those free from attachments can attain a vision of the unmanifest. Those who cling to attachments only perceive the outer form. To those who understand, the manifest and unmanifest are essentially one reality that differs only in name. This unity is the incomprehensible mystery that envelops existence.

As she attempts to grasp the meaning of those words, I am in the presence of the sage who authored them. He is seated by the bristlecone tree in the golden meadow under the golden sky.

"Hello, dear friends, I am Laozi and welcome to the Heavenly Meadow. This peaceful abode is a place of unlearning." Laozi picks up a white porcelain cup and pours tea into it. Steam wafts from the rim and he takes a sip. "Ahhh, delicious."

"May our time together empty your cups," he says as he pours the tea on the ground. "Most of you are asleep and one of you is deceased. Who is it that dreams across life and death, I wonder? Who is dreaming the world? Who is dreaming you? Those who abide in Dao know the unknowable truth. They have poured the tea from the cup of their head. Emptiness is the dreamer of all dreams. How could it be otherwise?

"The invisible hand of Dao has brought us together and each one of you is here for a reason, whether or not you know it." Laozi directs his gaze at a pale-faced man with a thick, unkempt mustache and blue eyes. "You over here, sir, kindly introduce yourself."

"My name is Clay and I lived in Iowa my entire life until I died. I guess I'm the dead guy in the group."

"How can you be so sure that you are dead and not dreaming?" Laozi asks as his eyes widen and his brows lifts.

"I'm pretty sure that I'm dead, but now that you mention it, maybe I'm dreaming that I'm dead," Clay replies.

"Rest assured, Clay, you're no longer alive. Tell us, dear friend, were the mysteries of existence revealed to you when you died?"

"Not really, sir. I kind of just woke up here."

"Did you become enlightened when you died?"

"No sir, I'm just about the same old Clay that I was, but maybe a little smarter on account of listening to folks like you lecture on these subjects."

"What brings you to Heavenly Meadow?" Laozi asks.

"Some of my friends were discussing your book," Clay said. "They were quoting it, and they were rambling on about this Dao thing and it sounded interesting, but I didn't really understand it. They struggled to make me understand. One of them advised that I should spend some time with you, and here I am."

"And what is your name?" Laozi asks a young man with a bright smile under a mop of disheveled hair.

"Tommy. And I read your book The Dao De Jing twice, and it's cool. I'm not sure I totally get the Dao either. And I'm asleep because I fell asleep reading it. And I would say that the Dao is something we can't see with our eyes. And it has no name. So, it's a mystery."

Laozi strokes his beard. "Thank you, Tommy. And Madame, what is your name?" Laozi asks a Black woman with a sizable tuft of braided hair knotted on her head.

"My name is Hadiza, Mister Laozi," she replies.

"And where are you from, Hadiza?"

"My body is currently asleep in my room in Stone Town, on the island of Zanzibar off the coast of Tanzania, in Africa. I also fell asleep reading your book."

"And Hadiza, in your opinion, what is Dao?"

"I was thinking about that very question when I dozed off. I am a religious woman, and I believe in God. Dao sounds a lot like God but without the personality. In the Koran there are many stories about God. In the Bible there are many stories about God. In your book, Dao has no stories. There are no prophets. The Dao is nameless and invisible. I imagine that the Dao is hard to worship. How can you pray to something that is so elusive and unlike a human being? How do you worship such a God?"

"Would it be easier for you to worship Dao if Dao was merciful and compassionate?" Laozi asks.

"Yes, of course. Those are the qualities of God. We seek the blessing of God. Especially when we are suffering and humbled by life. People become religious when they are most desperate. That is when we pray deepest. But how can one pray to this Dao? This was my question while I was falling asleep."

"What about you, sir? What is your name?" Laozi asks a rotund man with a helmet of short black hair cropped around a pair of small ears.

"My name is Marty. I live in Queens, New York. I manage a car dealership. I get my customers the best deal on the finest cars. My wife nags me about you all the time. She worships you and tells me to read your book. She bought me a copy for my birthday, but I'm not interested in books. I like sports. I like the thrill of my teams winning. The Yankees, the Jets, Knicks, the Rangers. Nothing is better than winning. So, her birthday comes, and I ask her what she wants. She says she wants us to read a chapter out loud together before bed for a week. And I agreed just to shut her up. So, we read a chapter tonight and I got to be honest, I'm not interested like I said, so I don't know what I'm doing here."

"If you're here, it's because you *are* interested," Laozi replies.

"Maybe I was a little curious about one thing. People at work, they don't like me too much," Marty says. "They say I'm a little rough around the edges. But I like it that way. I push them to produce. Money, money, money makes the world go round. If I scare them a little here and there, it's because they're slacking off. And sometimes, you just must keep people on guard, you know what I mean? My father taught me that it's a concrete jungle out there, so I might as well be the apex predator at the top of the food chain. The king of the mountain. I never understood this business of being meek and inheriting the earth. It sounds like a marketing scheme to attract suckers and get them to give you their money. But you wrote something about water being stronger than everything and that got me thinking. Because I would have thought that I'd rather be the mountain than the water that erodes it. So maybe that's why I woke up here."

"I'm very, very interested in everything you have to say," the woman sitting next to Marty blurts out. She has brown hair and black-rimmed glasses that enlarge her eyes. Exaggerated hand gestures accompany her speeding voice. "I've always been attracted to Daoism, and I even have a tattoo of a Yin and Yang symbol on my spine where I can't see it unless I look in the mirror. And I think that's what Dao is like. It's there all the time but it can't be seen unless you look for it where it can't be seen."

"What is your name?" Laozi asks.

"My name is Miranda and I'm sleeping in Kalamazoo. I'm so excited to be here."

"What is your profession, Miranda?"

"I am a librarian. I like to read a lot. I read three books a week, sometimes more. I love a good story. Fantasy, science fiction. I especially enjoy reading books about ancient religions and magic. I came across your book a long time ago. I don't remember how long ago. I must have been in my twenties. I still have the book on my bookshelf, and I pulled it out earlier this evening and read a few pages, and I still love it as much as I did the first time I read it. It's so mysterious and deep."

"And you, sir, what is your name?" Laozi asks.

"My name is Professor Fogarty, sir. I am a philosophy professor." The professor clears his voice and adds, "I teach classical Chinese and my class is currently reading your book. My interest in your work is academic. Earlier this evening I was grading essays. The topic of the essay was, coincidentally, 'What is the Dao?' and one student handed in a blank sheet of paper, and I spent the evening deliberating whether to grade her an F or an A. I fell asleep wondering, what you would do? I suppose I woke up here for that reason."

"I would give her an A plus," Tommy says.

"She deserves an F," Marty replies. "She's just being a bit too clever and a lot too lazy."

"What is your name?" Laozi asks a petite woman with blonde bangs covering her forehead and partially hanging over her blue eyes.

"My name is Astrid and I'm in New York City for a weekend workshop about Daoist meditation. It starts in a few hours, and I am very excited. I practice yoga and meditate every day. I have always been curious about Daoist practices, and I fell asleep wondering about you."

"Astrid, what does Dao mean to you?"

"I think it means everything that's good. Like love and charity, and wisdom, and longevity. It's about becoming positive and healthy. It's about getting rid of everything bad and negative. It's the ultimate in chill. That's what I think. But what do I know. See, I'm emptying my cup. I would love to hear what you have to say, Laozi."

Laozi nods and closes his eyes. His presence withdraws and his composure returns as his lids reopen. "The relative world is defined by opposition. Beauty defines ugly. Good defines evil. Easy defines difficult. Low defines high. Before defines after. The world is a circle of oppositions in relationship to each other like the spokes of a wheel. The spokes unite at the hub of the wheel. The emptiness on which they center allows the carriage wheel to be of use. The emptiness of the wheel defines the usefulness of the wheel. Glass is molded into a vessel. The emptiness of the glass defines its usefulness. The emptiness between the walls define the usefulness of a room. The emptiness between notes defines the music. Without emptiness, can there be anything? Without formlessness, can there be form? This emptiness lies at the center of all things. This emptiness presided before heaven and earth. This emptiness is the nonbeing at the heart of being. This emptiness is beyond measure, immutable, all pervading, inexhaustible, and nameless. Ask me to name it; I name it Dao—the Way."

"And what is your name?" Laozi asks a woman with a brown ponytail and a rosy complexion.

"My name is Sofia, and I am a park ranger in Colorado. I have always loved nature and I made a rewarding career out of doing what I can to keep our parks safe, as well as the animals who live in the park, and the people who visit. A few years ago, I overheard some people speaking at a coffee shop about your book and the importance that you place on human nature aligning with nature. I bought a copy and read it. I was intrigued. I was particularly drawn to the idea that human beings embody the mystery of their own existence, and that this mystery can be understood by going deep within.

"I found some practical books on Daoist meditation and began to practice at home. I couldn't believe it when I felt energy moving inside of me. I felt like an explorer who discovered a new continent. How come this knowledge isn't part of the public domain? Why aren't these practices taught to teenagers? These simple meditations were so deeply healing. I tracked down a teacher and I was lucky to find someone who lives a few towns over. I began to practice with him and his group, and my practice became deeper and more meaningful. The more I meditated, the more I wanted to meditate. I became a happier and more serene version of myself.

"And then, one day, everything changed. I was practicing an exercise that involved spinning energies in the area behind my navel, and suddenly, something deep inside me clicked and a doorway opened up. I experienced a new kind of energy flowing into me. This energy covered me like a cloud. And inside this cloud, I felt so peaceful. I opened my eyes to make sure the room was still there. I saw my teacher and the other students meditating and I closed my eyes and returned to the cloud. I felt a peacefulness that I had never experienced before. I felt so serene. It was perfection and my mind stopped moving. I was perfectly at peace. I experienced stillness. I didn't want to move. I could have stayed in that place forever.

"A few days passed, and I began to notice that my body was transforming. My body lost its usual feeling of heaviness and physicality. I became a body of energy and light. My muscles, blood, and bones were still there but they were permeated by a spaciousness that went on forever in all directions. If I brought my attention to the center of my head, I would lose myself in the spaciousness that opened. Meditation has become effortless. The experience of my own being is deepening, and every day is a blessing. I am happy to be alive and I am grateful for every moment of every day. I fell asleep this evening wanting to thank you. I guess that is the reason I am here."

"You are welcome, my dear child."

"Wow, that is so cool. It makes me want to wake up and start practicing right away," Tommy says. "Laozi, do you think that everyone can learn to meditate and feel that way?"

"Follow the Way of Virtue. This path leads back to the origin of your being. Follow the Dao of Virtue and you will attain perfect peace. Dao is open to all, Tommy."

"Thanks. Laozi, I promise you that I will!" Tommy exclaims.

"And you, sir, what is your name?" Laozi asks me.

Though I am eager to speak, the golden sky of Heavenly Meadow flickers and Laozi's face grows faint. Before I can speak a word, the Golden Meadow of Laozi is vanishing. The last thing I see are his eyes as I feel the mattress moving under me and I hear a stretch and yawn.

"Good morning, Robert," my wife Dongmei says.

"Good morning," I reply.

She draws the curtain and light streams in.

"Oh, look at this. It's a beautiful day," Dongmei says. "Did you sleep well?"

"I had an unusual dream," I reply.

"Tell me about it at breakfast. I'm hungry."

"Sure."

"Why don't we go for a walk after our morning meditation?"

"Good idea," I reply, wondering what they are discussing in Heavenly Meadow, hoping to return sometime soon.

Acknowledgments for Robert Peng

I would like to express my heartfelt appreciation to all the individuals whose invaluable help and unwavering support made a profound difference during the process of writing this book.

First and foremost, my deepest gratitude goes to my beloved wife, Dongmei, whose love, support, knowledge, and clear vision have been instrumental in shaping this book. Her encouragement to turn my years of individual practice into a comprehensive course proved to be a wonderful suggestion, and her insightful advice on the book's content and structure was highly valuable.

I must also extend my sincere acknowledgment to my coauthor and brother, Rafael Nasser. Like in the first book, *The Master Key*, Rafi has made significant contributions to every aspect of this book—from its overall structure to the writing of each chapter, and in helping develop the beautiful illustrations within. His vast knowledge, talent, wisdom, and exceptional writing skills have transformed my teachings into the beautiful book you hold in your hands. I am also deeply grateful to his wife, Sandra, and son, Gabriel, for their generous support and love.

I extend my sincere thanks and credit to Tobin Dorn, whose artistic talent and illustrations have transformed each image into a work of art that captures the essence of energy work. My appreciation also goes to Evan Lui for his professional photography skills. To my students and friends who modeled for the illustrations: Alejandra Cohen, Ishmael Cato, and Ellen Petersen. I am grateful for their devotion and inner peace, which are vividly portrayed in the illustrations.

Special thanks to Jessica Carew Kraft, who helped shape my workshop into the foundational structure of this book. I am filled with gratitude for Kenneth Cohen and Patty de Llosa, who provided valuable comments on the book.

I am indebted to Jon Gabriel Abrams for his wise counsel, and to Deborah Boyar for her selfless contributions of feedback and editing. Special thanks to The Love Studio for the photo shoot, and I am also grateful to Eric Yang, Carole Donahoe, and Veronica Domingo for their valuable suggestions regarding the models and photographer.

I would like to also extend my deepest gratitude to Sounds True and the entire team for their invaluable support and guidance in the creation of this book. Your expertise, dedication, and passion have been instrumental in bringing this project to fruition. Thank you for your commitment to publishing works that enlighten and inspire.

Lastly, I want to express my heartfelt thanks to my family members and friends, as well as to all my students worldwide, for their continued encouragement and goodwill. Without each and every one of you, this book would not have been possible. Your support has been a driving force behind this work. Thank you from the bottom of my heart.

Acknowledgments for Rafael Nasser

Working on *The Way of Virtue* has been an honor and a privilege for which I am grateful. Robert, thank you for your brotherly friendship and for trusting me to help your wisdom find a voice. My contribution to this book is dedicated to my son, Gabriel, a toddler wise beyond his years. I thank my wife, Sandra, for her love and support. I also wish to thank the following people who enriched my spiritual life with their wisdom and friendship:

Ayala Ashear, Amnon Shiboleth, Barbara Larisch, Christian Kurz, Rabbi David Ingber, Deborah Boyar, Donald Abrams, Dongmei Liu, Elaine Thomas, Sifu Frank Matos, Fransje, Gia Caspi, Reverend Gregory Kehn, Swami Hariharananda, Harry Nasser, Ishmael Cato, Dr. Issam Nemeh and family, John Marchesella, Jon Abrams, Julia March, Julia Raether, Karinna Karsten, Lloyd Abrams, Magaly Blakz, Michael Winn, Mitchell Rabin, Nancy Packes, Neil Sonenberg, Neri Baron, Robert Gehorsam, Sierra Abrams, Steven Forrest, Dr. Steve Jackowicz, Steve Nadel, The Celestial Sisters, Tim Klemt, Tobin Dorn our talented designer, Victoria Bernstein, and Yael Melamed.

About the Authors

Robert Peng was born in Hunan Province, China. As a young boy, he met a monk named Xiao Yao who became his spiritual guide. Robert trained daily with his teacher for years in the healing arts of Qigong and meditation. At the age of fifteen, Robert embarked on an extraordinary hundred-day water fast in a dark stone chamber below the temple hall of a secluded mountaintop monastery. This remarkable experience catalyzed a deep spiritual transformation and awakened healing abilities within him.

After graduating from Zhongnan University with a degree in English, Robert began to teach Qigong to a group of students and professors. His reputation grew and his teachings attracted the attention of thousands of students. Eventually, Robert migrated to Australia and then to the United States, spreading his Qigong knowledge worldwide. In recent years, Robert also started teaching online classes aiming to make Qigong's wisdom universally accessible.

Robert has authored two books with his friend and student Rafael Nasser. *The Master Key: Qigong Secrets for Vitality, Love, and Wisdom* details his autobiography and presents the foundational building blocks of the system he teaches. *The Way of Virtue: Qigong Meditations to Achieve Perfect Peace in an Imperfect World* describes the nature of the mind and guides the reader toward the awakening of Spirit.

Currently, Robert lives in Hudson Valley, New York, with his wife, Dongmei.

Rafael Nasser met Robert Peng in 2005. This serendipitous connection blossomed into a mentorship that went beyond imparting the discipline of Qigong. Together, they embarked on creating *The Master Key: Qigong Secrets for Vitality, Love, and Wisdom* and more recently *The Way of Virtue: Qigong Meditations to Achieve Perfect Peace in an Imperfect World*. These collaborative works reflect Rafael's deep appreciation of Qigong and his shared passion with Robert for transmitting the wisdom of this ancient spiritual artform in lucid language that stirs the modern soul. Rafael lives in bucolic New England, surrounded by serene beauty and inspiring silence that sustains his exploration of consciousness.

About Sounds True

Sounds True was founded in 1985 by Tami Simon with a clear mission: to disseminate spiritual wisdom. Since starting out as a project with one woman and her tape recorder, we have grown into a multimedia publishing company with a catalog of more than 3,000 titles by some of the leading teachers and visionaries of our time, and an ever-expanding family of beloved customers from across the world.

In more than three decades of evolution, Sounds True has maintained our focus on our overriding purpose and mission: to wake up the world. We offer books, audio programs, online learning experiences, and in-person events to support your personal growth and awakening, and to unlock our greatest human capacities to love and serve.

At SoundsTrue.com you'll find a wealth of resources to enrich your journey, including our weekly *Insights at the Edge* podcast, free downloads, and information about our nonprofit Sounds True Foundation, where we strive to remove financial barriers to the materials we publish through scholarships and donations worldwide.

To learn more, please visit SoundsTrue.com/freegifts or call us toll-free at 800.333.9185.

Together, we can wake up the world.

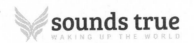